PLACEBO EFFECTS IN SPORT AND EXERCISE

Placebo effects have been recognised by medicine and by science, yet only recently has systematic research begun to fully understand what they are and how they work. Sport and exercise scientists started systematic research to better understand the potential performance-enhancing effects of placebos as well as how a range of treatments are used in sport, from nutritional supplements to psychological interventions to sports medicine treatments. *Placebo Effects in Sport and Exercise* synthesises this field of research of the influence placebo effects have in sport and exercise.

This book brings together many of the world's leading and emerging placebo effect researchers to help readers gain an understanding of core research findings from within sports and exercise science as well as sport and exercise-related contributions from experts in anthropology, medicine, and neuroscience. Readers will gain an insight of what placebo and nocebo effects are, how they might influence sport and exercise performance and outcomes, and how they might significantly influence the effectiveness of performance and health interventions.

The book investigates various practical and ethical implications for the sport and exercise practitioner, student, and researcher to consider. Can a placebo work if the athlete knows it's a placebo? Should practitioners use placebos to enhance performance? Can the use of placebos reduce doping? Are some sports medicine treatments little more than placebos?

With the rapid growth of applied sports medicine, as well as the concept of exercise as a mental health treatment in its own right, *Placebo Effects in Sport and Exercise* is key reading for students and researchers of sport psychology as well as those out in the field.

Philip Hurst, PhD, is a Senior Lecturer in Sport and Exercise Psychology at the School of Psychology and Life Sciences at Canterbury Christ Church University, UK.

Chris Beedie is an Honorary Professor and an affiliate of the Cognition and Neuroscience Research Group at the School of Psychology at the University of Kent, UK.

PLACEBO EFFECTS IN SPORT AND EXERCISE

Edited by Philip Hurst and Chris Beedie

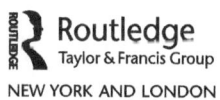
Routledge
Taylor & Francis Group

NEW YORK AND LONDON

Designed cover image: Getty Images

First published 2024
by Routledge
605 Third Avenue, New York, NY 10158

and by Routledge
4 Park Square, Milton Park, Abingdon, Oxon, OX14 4RN

Routledge is an imprint of the Taylor & Francis Group, an informa business

ISBN: 978-1-032-13395-9 (hbk)
ISBN: 978-1-032-13394-2 (pbk)
ISBN: 978-1-003-22900-1 (ebk)

DOI: 10.4324/9781003229001

Typeset in Galliard
by SPi Technologies India Pvt Ltd (Straive)

CONTENTS

List of illustrations   *viii*
List of contributors   *x*

1 What are placebo effects? An introduction   1
  John S. Raglin

2 Can placebo effects go wrong? The nocebo effect in
  sport and exercise   11
  Luana Colloca

3 Can a placebo effect make me faster? Evidence for
  placebo effects as performance enhancers in sport   23
  *Guilherme Matta, Florentina Hettinga, and
  Andrew Edwards*

4 What happens in my brain when I experience a placebo
  effect? Neurobiological mechanisms of placebo effects   35
  Bart Roelands

5 Are placebo effects special? A social-evolutionary
  perspective on resource perception in exercise-induced
  fatigue and performance   45
  Emma Cohen

6 Do I think or do I feel a placebo effect? Placebo effects
   and emotion in sport   57
   Chris Beedie

7 Are placebo effects a perceptual illusion? Placebo effects
   on performance within the Bayesian Brain   72
   *Aaron Greenhouse-Tucknott, Jake B. Butterworth,
   James G. Wrightson, and Jeanne Dekerle*

8 Can we replace oxygen, at least partially, with a placebo?
   Placebo effects at high altitude   85
   Fabrizio Benedetti

9 Can we remove placebo effects from exercise
   interventions? Methodological considerations for
   understanding the psychological benefits of exercise   99
   Jacob B. Lindheimer

10 Do placebo effects improve my skill? The influence of
   placebo effects on motor control and learning   113
   Mirta Fiorio and Diletta Barbiani

11 How do I use placebo effects to improve my
   interventions? Harnessing knowledge of placebo effects
   to maximise the effectiveness of interventions in sport   123
   Andrew M. Lane, Ross Cloak, and Tracey J. Devonport

12 Do you have to lie to induce placebo effects? The use of
   open label placebos in sport and exercise   133
   *Bryan Saunders, Felipe Miguel Marticorena, and
   Bruno Gualano*

13 If I inject words not drugs, will athletes be less likely
   to dope?   144
   Philip Hurst and Abby Foad

14 Is it OK to recommend complementary or alternative
   medicine even though I know it's a placebo? Why the
   neurobiology of the placebo effect does not legitimise
   the use of CAM   156
   Chris Beedie

15 Can I use the placebo effect to treat injured or ill
   athletes? Ethics, deception, and placebo effects in sports
   medicine   169
   Marcus Campos, Pascal Borry, and Mike McNamee

Index   *182*

ILLUSTRATIONS

Figures

1.1 A psychosocial model of the placebo effect in the context of sport (from: Raglin et al. 2020) 6

7.1 The foundation of generative models of the world following Bayes' theorem 74

7.2 The proposed effect of placebo on pain ratings based on Bayesian theory 78

8.1 General subdivision of different altitude zones, and the altitudes where we have data about placebo effects (3500 m, 4500 m, 5500 m) 87

8.2 Four physiological functions (ventilation, oxygenation, circulation, perfusion), along with physical performance, have been investigated by recording several physiological parameters 90

8.3 The effects of placebo given for the first time, of oxygen, and of placebo after oxygen preconditioning on minute ventilation, blood pH, heart rate, PGE2, headache, fatigue at 3500 m 91

8.4 Here performance is measured as the time needed to complete 3000 steps on a stepper 94

9.1 Distinguishing the true effect of exercise on psychological responses from non-specific effects requires the inclusion of a placebo and no-treatment control group 101

11.1 Proposed model of working with beliefs effects when delivering interventions 129

12.1   The four main discussion points to be discussed with the
       individual during the open-label placebo intervention,
       namely that i) placebo effects are powerful; ii) the body
       may automatically respond to taking placebo pills similar to
       Pavlov's dogs; iii) a positive attitude helps; and iv) taking the
       pills is a critical component   134
12.2   The efficacy of the open-label placebo intervention may
       depend upon the information provided   137

Tables

7.1   Glossary of terms used within predictive processing   76
9.1   The balanced placebo design is a model for observing
      expectancy-related placebo effects that can be adapted
      to studying psychological responses to exercise if a valid
      exercise placebo is ever developed   107
13.1 Key topics, aims and tasks that facilitators can use to embed
      into anti-doping interventions   149

CONTRIBUTORS

Diletta Barbiani
Department of Neurosciences,
    Biomedicine and Movement
    Sciences
University of Verona
Verona, Italy
and
Department of Psychology
Università Cattolica del Sacro Cuore,
Milan, Italy

Chris Beedie
Department of Psychology
University of Kent
Canterbury, UK

Fabrizio Benedetti
Department of Neuroscience
University of Turin Medical School
Turin, Italy
and
Hypoxia Medicine and Physiology
Plateau Rosà, Switzerland

Pascal Borry
Department of Public Health
KU Leuven
Leuven, Belgium

Jake B. Butterworth
Fatigue and Exercise Laboratory
School of Sport and Health
    Sciences
University of Brighton
Brighton, East Sussex, UK

Marcus Campos
Department of Movement Sciences
and
Department of Public Health and
    Primary Care
KU Leuven
Leuven, Belgium

Ross Cloak
Faculty of Education, Health and
    Wellbeing
University of Wolverhampton
Wolverhampton, UK

Emma Cohen
Institute of Human Sciences
and
Wadham College
University of Oxford
Oxford, UK

Luana Colloca
Department of Pain and
  Translational Symptom Science
and
Placebo Beyond Opinions Center
School of Nursing
University of Maryland
Baltimore, Maryland, USA

Jeanne Dekerle
Fatigue and Exercise Laboratory
School of Sport and Health Sciences
University of Brighton
Brighton, East Sussex, UK

Tracey J. Devonport
Sport and Physical Activity Research
  Center
University of Wolverhampton
Wolverhampton, UK

Andrew Edwards
School of Psychology and Life
  Sciences
and
Science, Engineering and Social
  Sciences
Canterbury Christ Church
  University
Canterbury, UK

Mirta Fiorio
Department of Neurosciences,
  Biomedicine and Movement
  Sciences
University of Verona
Verona, Italy

Abby Foad
Centre for Sport, Physical Education
  and Activity Research
Canterbury Christ Church
  University
Canterbury, UK

Aaron Greenhouse-Tucknott
Fatigue and Exercise Laboratory
School of Sport and Health
  Sciences
University of Brighton
Brighton, East Sussex, UK

Bruno Gualano
Applied Physiology and Nutrition
  Research Group
School of Physical Education and
  Sport
Rheumatology Division
Faculdade de Medicina FMUSP
and
Lifestyle Medicine Center
University of São Paulo
São Paulo, Brazil

Florentina Hettinga
Department of Sport, Exercise and
  Rehabilitation
Faculty of Health and Life Sciences
Northumbria University
Newcastle upon Tyne, UK

Philip Hurst
School of Psychology and Life
  Sciences
Canterbury Christ Church
  University
Canterbury, UK

Andrew M. Lane
Faculty of Education, Health and
  Wellbeing
University of Wolverhampton
Wolverhampton, UK

Jacob B. Lindheimer
Department of Veterans Affairs
William S. Middleton Veterans
  Memorial Hospital
Madison, Wisconsin, USA

Guilherme Matta
School of Psychology and Life
  Sciences
Faculty of Science, Engineering and
  Social Sciences
Canterbury Christ Church
  University
Canterbury, UK

Mike McNamee
Faculty of Movement and
  Rehabilitation Sciences
KU Leuven
Leuven, Belgium
and
School of Sport and Exercise Sciences
Swansea University
Swansea, Wales, UK

Felipe Miguel Marticorena
Applied Physiology and Nutrition
  Research Group
School of Physical Education and
  Sport
Rheumatology Division
Faculdade de Medicina FMUSP
University of São Paulo
São Paulo, Brazil

John S. Raglin
Department of Kinesiology
Indiana University
Bloomington, Indiana, USA

Bart Roelands
Human Physiology and Sports
  Physiotherapy Research Group
Vrije Universiteit Brussel
Brussels, Belgium

Bryan Saunders
Applied Physiology and Nutrition
  Research Group
School of Physical Education and
  Sport
Rheumatology Division
and
Institute of Orthopaedics and
  Traumatology
Faculty of Medicine FMUSP
University of São Paulo
São Paulo, Brazil

James G. Wrightson
University of British Columbia
Vancouver, British Columbia,
  Canada

1

WHAT ARE PLACEBO EFFECTS?

An introduction

John S. Raglin

Introduction

The term Placebo – which in Latin translates as "I will please" – first appeared in Psalm 116:9 in the 14th-century Latin Bible was actually a mistranslation of the Hebrew for "I will walk" (Evans, 2003; Shapiro, 1968). Soon after the term was used during the rise of the Black Death to describe hired as mourners at funerals to fill in family members who had also succumbed to the plague or were understandably absent. Subsequently, the term evolved into a common insult to describe feigned sincerity.

The association of the term 'placebo' with medicine is generally believed to have begun in the 18th century, but examples have been traced back more than a millennia earlier to the writings of Galen (Guijarro, 2015). The most celebrated historical application of a placebo to evaluate a medical intervention also preceded its first appearance in a medical text. In 1784, Benjamin Franklin and several other distinguished scientists, including Antoine Lavoisier, were commissioned by King Louis XVI to investigate the controversial medical practices of the physician Franz Mesmer. Mesmer had become a *cause célèbre* among his wealthy Parisian patients by treating them for various maladies using "animal magnetism," an invisible force he claimed to have discovered. Franklin's commission utilised what is now regarded as the first placebo control, although it was not described as such in their report. They compared the effects of objects treated with animal magnetism ("mesmerised") with untreated objects on patients who had previous experience with mesmerism, and in some tests the patients wore blindfolds to prevent them from identifying the treatment they were receiving. Their findings revealed that the patients responded similarly whether exposed to mesmerised or untreated objects, and

DOI: 10.4324/9781003229001-1

the commission concluded the effects of Mesmerism were solely a consequence of "imagination".. In a correspondence that predated the commission's work, Franklin (Franklin, 1784) attributed the benefits of similarly dubious medical practices to "expectation", consistent with current perspectives on placebo mechanisms. The commission's use of a variant of the single-blind placebo control – wherein participants do not know whether or not they are receiving the actual treatment – has since been regarded as a major innovation in scientific investigation, but it is not without precedent. For example, two centuries earlier the Catholic church evaluated the effectiveness of exorcisms by comparing responses to holy objects or unblessed equivalents (Kaptchuk et al., 2009).

The first medical definition of the placebo effect in a textbook also occurred in the late 18th century (Shapiro, 1968), although it has been more widely ascribed to a medical dictionary published in 1811 in which a placebo was described as "an epithet given to any medicine adapted more to please than to benefit the patient" (Quincy, 1811, p. 684). This description remained largely unchanged for well over a century when Beecher (1955) substituted "epithet" with "pharmacologically inert substances" in his 1955 review of the medical literature on placebos. Of far greater impact was Beecher's claim that placebos benefitted an overall average 35.2% of patients suffering from various medical conditions, an assertion that many feel initiated the current era of scientific scrutiny of the placebo effect as a legitimate phenomenon.

Up to this point in the history of the placebo effect, that is the late 1950s, it was almost entirely associated with medicine and the treatment of the ailing patient, not the healthy and vigorous athlete. A rare exception was an ambitious investigation of the ergogenic effects of amphetamine on athletes published by Beecher and colleagues several years following his influential review (Smith & Beecher, 1959, 1960). The study utilised not only double-blind placebo controls, but also several other innovations that remain rarely incorporated in sport placebo research to this day. These included self-report assessments of the athlete's expectations of the treatments and their side effects, tests involving different sports and events within a single sport occurring in either a competitive and non-competitive setting. The results were widely cited in sports magazines but failed to stimulate further research in sports, perhaps in part because of criticisms of its data collection methods and statistical analyses (Hollister, 1960; Pierson, 1961).

Criticism of statistical methods continued to shadow the medical placebo literature long after Beecher's paper. Foremost among them was the potential contribution of "non-specific effects" (Kienle & Kiene, 1997; Roberts, 1995) that were falsely attributed to placebos. Although the concept is not without its critics (Peek, 1977), non-specific effects refer to reductions in the symptoms of a disease that may also result in a favourable change in its status (i.e., ill, remised, cured) which occur with the passage of time, whether or not the patient received an active treatment or placebo. The most commonly described examples are regression toward the mean, spontaneous improvement, and the natural fluctuation or natural history of symptoms (Kienle & Kiene, 1997). Quantifying the impact of non-specific effects in an experiment requires the addition of a non-treatment control arm, a condition absent in many placebo studies (Kienle & Kiene, 1997; see also Chapter 9). Non-specific effects have also been commonly cited as the basis for placebo effects in sport performance studies, but it has been noted (Lindheimer et al., in press) that these would either be absent in the context of sport as in the case of spontaneous remission, or they would result in impaired rather than improved performance as in the case of regression toward the mean. Other critiques have attributed placebo effects to a rise in motivation, but this is unlikely, particularly for elite athletes who already score extremely high on standardised measures of motivation. As in the case in medicine, many sport scientists have simply dismissed the placebo effect entirely, decrying it as illusory or imagined.

In recent years, however, such criticisms or dismissals of the placebo effect have been subverted by the findings of innovative research that has employed brain imaging technology to examine the neurobiological activity during placebo administration. Another innovation is the use of novel designs that extend beyond the randomised control trial (RCT) to assess the influence of expectation and conditioning of placebo treatments, such as the balanced placebo design, open-hidden designs, graded expectations, and open label studies.

The findings of this research reveal that placebos often work by activating the same neurobiological pathways as the medication they purport to be, yielding real benefits that add to the efficacy of proven treatments though expectation and conditioning. Relatedly, studies involving manipulated or graded expectations in which the likelihood of receiving a treatment is raised (e.g., 75%) or lowered (e.g., 25%) have found that the strength of expectation can influence the efficacy of both placebos and actual treatments (Pollo et al., 2001), although these results have yet to be successfully replicated in a sports performance paradigm (Carlino et al., 2014). The implications of this body of findings are important for both research and clinical practice. For example, the RCT has long been deemed the gold standard for assessing the efficacy of a medical intervention by quantifying the independent contribution of placebos to treatment outcomes. However, the use of a double-blind control results in a conditional expectation in which the participant knows there is an equal chance (50–50) of receiving either the placebo or actual treatment, and it has been found that this 50% conditional expectation often reduces the efficacy of both the treatment and the placebo (Carlino et al., 2014). Moreover, in clinical settings not only is there a 100% expectation of receiving the actual treatment, but it is often paired with positive messages of effectiveness (e.g., "this is a powerful pain killer"), a combination that often results in enhanced efficacy. The contribution of expectation on both treatment and placebo efficacy can be assessed using the balanced-placebo design that incorporates conditions in which expectations are either 0% or 100% (see also Lindheimer's chapter in this book).

Definitions: Placebo, placebo effect, nocebo

Whether used in an experimental study or clinical practice or sport setting, a *placebo* is an inert agent or sham treatment that lacks any inherent biological, nutritional, or mechanical constituents capable of producing a biological or psychological benefit (Kirsch, 1985). Similarly, a *placebo effect* refers to any beneficial biological (e.g., reduced blood pressure) or psychological (e.g., reduced anxiety) outcome that can be attributed to the placebo, or occurs solely as a consequence of expectation or conditioning, the same processes by which placebos are established (Benedetti et al., 2003)which often are present in treatment conditions. This latter example indicates that placebo effects can occur in the absence of placebos, and there is research indicating that conditioning and expectation add to the efficacy of many active treatments, including pain medication (Benedetti et al., 2003). The term *placebo response* has been applied as a synonym for placebo effect but is more commonly used to describe changes due to non-specific effects (e.g., regression toward the mean) and potential experimental artifacts (e.g., demand characteristics) that occur during a clinical trial or research study. Accordingly, a non-treatment control condition would be needed to distinguish the placebo response from a true placebo effect.

Additional categories have been used to classify placebos. An *inert placebo* (sometimes called a pure placebo) uses ingredients that lack any pharmacological and physiological effects (e.g., an injection of saline solution or a capsule filled with corn powder). An *active placebo*, by contrast, is intentionally formulated to be more convincing by mimicking not only the physical appearance of the medication but also some of its sensory characteristics, such as smell or taste, or side effects. Studies have found that active placebos often yield greater effects compared with generic placebos (Miller & Colloca, 2009). Another reason to consider using active placebos is that many medical or ergogenic treatments have strong sensory characteristics (e.g., taste) or side effects (e.g., tachycardia) and their absence could alert participants that they are receiving a placebo rather than the active treatment, a phenomenon referred to as functional unblinding. For example, an athlete who was a regular user of creatine was able to determine he was given a placebo in a study because he failed to experience any of the typical gastric or hydration symptoms he typically experienced when taking creatine Chris Beedie (personal communication March 8 2023) described how an athlete reported knowing he had been allocated to the placebo control arm of a study of creatine, because having used creatine previously he expected certain gastric and hydration effects that were absent over the period of the study.

However, the circumstances in which the use of an active placebo would be more effective in blinding participants about the condition they have been assigned to are not easily predicted aforehand. For example, it would be anticipated that athletes who regularly used caffeine as an ergogenic aid would be less likely to be deceived by an inert placebo. Yet in a study (Saunders et al., 2017) comparing the benefits of caffeine pill against an inert placebo on cycling performance in competitive cyclists who regularly consumed it, only 40.4% correctly identified the placebo. Even when given the opportunity to change their response following the test, the percent of participants correctly identifying the placebo improved by only 7.2% to 47.6%. Conversely, there are cases in which participants can distinguish between convincingly designed active placebos from an active treatment that lacks overt sensory cues that could unveil the deceptive condition. In a study involving frequent tanning bed users (Feldman et al., 2004) who were given the choice to use either a UV bed or identical placebo bed that did not emit UV rays, only 5% of the participants chose the non-UV bed. These results, along with research finding stronger benefits when participants have a greater expectation of receiving the active treatment (e.g., 75% versus 25% or 50%), emphasise the importance of assessing the confidence that participants have about either receiving the active treatment or placebo (see also Chapter 11). This information could be used to conduct post hoc analyses in order to determine if the presence or absence of strong expectations in participants influenced their responses to either an experimental treatment or placebo during the intervention.

A final category that could be confused with the active placebo is the *impure placebo*, a medication or treatment with pharmacological or physiological outcomes, but which have no documented benefit on the patient's medical condition or symptoms either because it is administered at an ineffectively low dose or as an off-label medication. Despite this, the use of impure placebos is a surprisingly common practice (Fent et al., 2011; Chapter 14 and 15).

The administration of an inert medication or intervention presented with the expectation of negative outcomes (e.g., anxiety, pain, fatigue) may provoke negative symptoms or behaviors and is referred to as the *nocebo effect* ("I will harm"; Benedetti et al., 2003; Carlino et al., 2014). Sport scientists have proposed the following definition of a nocebo: "an inert ergogenic aid that is administered with the suggestion of a negative consequence on athletic performance" (Raglin et al., 2020; Chapter 2). Sport research has identified that the presentation of nocebos can worsen athletic performance, often to a far greater degree to that which placebos enhance it (Beedie et al., 2020; Beedie & Foad, 2009; Hurst et al., 2020). Inert agents presented in the absence of explicit messages of harm may still provoke nocebo effects among individuals who already possess negative expectations as a result of past experiences, knowledge or beliefs (i.e., habitual expectation); observe nocebo responses in others (i.e., social learning); or who develop negative expectations during the course of an experiment (i.e., incidentally-induced expectation). The latter can explain instances when placebos paradoxically induce a nocebo effect. In a study (Beedie et al., 2006) assessing the influence of placebo caffeine on cycling performance, a group of athletes were cued to expect a "substantial effect" from a large dose of caffeine that was actually a placebo. One participant who initially expected to perform well was unable to even complete the test after complaining about "feeling terrible" because of the side effects of the apparently high dose, 9 mg/kg, of caffeine. Paradoxically, there are cases in which unpleasant side effects associated with an ergogenic aid could exert a beneficial effect on performance. The athlete community is well aware of less palatable aspects of many ergogenic aids – "If it tastes bad it must be good for you" – and so unpleasant tastes or negative side effect may be perceived as evidence of potent ingredients, thereby generating positive expectations. Research has shown that that bitter tasting, but ergogenic inert drinks are associated with improved sport performance (Gam et al., 2016). A comprehensive understanding of placebo and nocebo effects must not only acknowledge that the characteristics of placebos influence their efficacy, but also recognise features of the psychosocial context in which they are administered (Benedetti, 2013). These include the role of the provider of the placebo (e.g., physician, therapist, or coach) and the setting in which the placebo is provided (e.g., hospital, clinic, or stadium). This has led researchers to broaden the definition of the placebo to acknowledge the influence of these factors. A recent iteration based on this perspective has been created for the context of sport in which a placebo is defined as: "the simulation of a proven ergogenic aid within a psychosocial context" (Raglin et al., 2020). A sport-oriented schematic of a psychosocial model of the placebo adapted from Benedetti (2013) is presented in Figure 1.1.

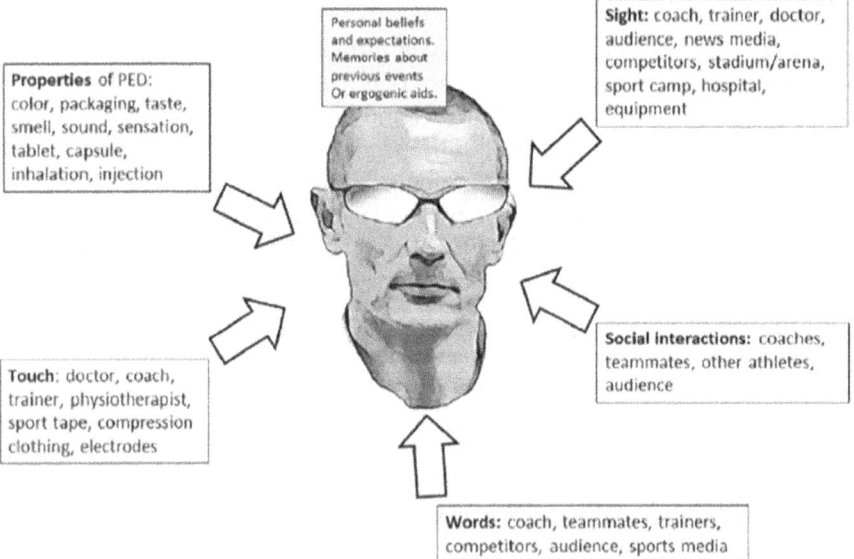

FIGURE 1.1 A psychosocial model of the placebo effect in the context of sport. (from: Raglin et al. 2020).

Processes leading to the formation of placebo effects: Expectation and conditioning

Expectation

Expectation is the primary process behind the establishment of placebo effects. Expectations have been described as predictions about future events (Kirsch, 1999) arising from existing experience, knowledge, or beliefs. Expectations can be modified by factors such as suggestion, observational learning, and conditioning. Some researchers have distinguished between expectations associated with stimuli or with responses. Kirsch (1999) has described stimulus expectancies as "anticipations of external events", and response expectancies as "predictions of nonvolitional responses". A stimulus expectation in the context of sport could involve the anticipated difficulty of a sporting event, whereas the response expectancy would be the expectation that the perceived exertion of the event will be lower or higher independent of performance. The term 'belief' has often been used synonymously with expectation, but many researchers regard them to be largely independent constructs (DeGood & Tait, 2001).

Conditioning

Placebo effects can also be established by classical conditioning. This occurs when an unconditioned stimulus (e.g., medication in a capsule) that evokes an unconditioned response (i.e., analgesia) becomes paired or associated with an unconditioned stimulus (i.e., the capsule itself). The unconditioned stimulus may include not only the capsule and its physical characteristics, such as size or color, but also the situational cues or sensory features, such as the smell of disinfectant, in the environment in which it was presented. These could include the treatment context (a hospital), or characteristics of the person administering the capsule (a clinician wearing a white coat). Following a sufficient number of presentations, the conditioned stimulus (i.e., the capsule) can result in analgesia (i.e., conditioned response) in the absence of any actual medication. Most researchers contend that classical conditioning-mediated placebo effects occur below the level of awareness and involve bodily changes that are not perceived (i.e., unconscious), but there is evidence that conditioning can change expectations (Meissner et al., 2011). Conversely, it has also been proposed that some expectations are non-conscious and so some researchers define conditioning as either explicit, resulting in conscious expectations or as implicit and non-conscious conditioning which does not generate expectations (Stewart-Williams & Podd, 2004). These findings reinforce the difficulty that can arise when attempting to determine what events led to the formation of a placebo effect.

Summary

Throughout its history, the placebo effect has been almost entirely conceptualised and studied from the perspective of medicine and the ailing patient. Sport-based studies with athletes were either ignored or regarded as a curious but incidental aspect of placebo research and theory. However, sport researchers have begun to utilise the same technological and methodological innovations that have revolutionised thinking about the placebo and its effects in medicine. The findings of their work have not only documented the contribution of placebo effects to sport performance but perhaps more importantly, added to the broader understanding of placebos and placebo mechanisms.

Research on the performance-enhancing effects of placebos has found that their ergogenic benefits result from the potentiation of the same neurobiological pathways as do placebos used in the context of medicine and illness. This indicates that placebos have the ability not just to alleviate the symptoms of patients suffering from medical conditions, but also to improve the functioning and performance of adults who exhibit superior health and physical conditioning. It is evident that some of these improvements stem from the reduction of pain or fatigue as do many medical placebos, but there are likely neurobiological processes which are unique to the context of sport. For instance, perception of exertion is often conflated with fatigue in the medical literature, but research indicates it is only moderately correlated with fatigue as well as pain,, and the sensation of exertion has been shown to involve unique neurobiological processes (Williamson et al., 2001). Additionally, high levels of felt energy or vigor are associated with superior athletic performance and aid in the resistance to sport maladies such as the overtraining syndrome (Raglin, 2007), and there is growing evidence these positive feelings are independent from and evoke different neurological activity than those associated with fatigue (Dishman et al., 2010; Loy et al., 2018). Finally, consistent with research involving medical placebos, athletes exhibit considerable individual differences in their responses to placebos. Information revealing that athletes are either similar or different from participants in medical studies in respect of the characteristics that influence placebo or nocebo responsiveness would enhance our general understanding of the placebo effect, and potentially lead to more effective practices in enhancing placebo effects in clinical practice.

The growth in scope and sophistication of sport placebo research has begun to draw from the periphery into the mainstream of the general field of placebo studies. It is now evident that many of the unanswered questions about sport placebos will have important implications to our greater theoretical understanding of placebos and their potential applications in clinical practice.

References

Beecher, H. K. (1955). The powerful placebo. *Journal of the American Medical Association, 159*(17), 1602–1606.

Beedie, C., Benedetti, F., Barbiani, D., Camerone, E., Lindheimer, J., & Roelands, B. (2020). Incorporating methods and findings from neuroscience to better understand placebo and nocebo effects in sport. *European Journal of Sport Science, 20*(3), 313–325.

Beedie, C. J., & Foad, A. J. (2009). The placebo effect in sports performance: A brief review. *Sports Medicine, 39*, 313–329.

Beedie, C. J., Stuart, E. M., Coleman, D. A., & Foad, A. J. (2006). Placebo effects of caffeine on cycling performance. *Medicine and Science in Sports and Exercise, 38*(12), 2159.

Benedetti, F. (2013). Placebo and the new physiology of the doctor-patient relationship. *Physiological Reviews, 93*(3), 1207–1246.

Benedetti, F., Pollo, A., Lopiano, L., Lanotte, M., Vighetti, S., & Rainero, I. (2003). Conscious expectation and unconscious conditioning in analgesic, motor, and hormonal placebo/nocebo responses. *Journal of Neuroscience, 23*(10), 4315–4323.

Carlino, E., Piedimonte, A., & Frisaldi, E. (2014). The effects of placebos and nocebos on physical performance. *Placebo*, 149–157.

DeGood, D. E., & Tait, R. C. (2001). Assessment of pain beliefs and pain coping. In D. Turk & R. Melzack (Eds.), *Handbook of pain assessment*. The Guilford Press.

Dishman, R. K., Thom, N. J., Puetz, T. W., O'Connor, P. J., & Clementz, B. A. (2010). Effects of cycling exercise on vigor, fatigue, and electroencephalographic activity among young adults who report persistent fatigue. *Psychophysiology, 47*(6), 1066–1074.

Evans, D. (2003). *Placebo: The belief effect*. HarperCollins London.

Feldman, S. R., Liguori, A., Kucenic, M., Rapp, S. R., Fleischer Jr, A. B., Lang, W., & Kaur, M. (2004). Ultraviolet exposure is a reinforcing stimulus in frequent indoor tanners. *Journal of the American Academy of Dermatology, 51*(1), 45–51.

Fent, R., Rosemann, T., Fässler, M., Senn, O., & Huber, C. A. (2011). The use of pure and impure placebo interventions in primary care-a qualitative approach. *BMC Family Practice, 12*(1), 1–7.

Franklin, B. (1784). *The papers of Benjamin Franklin: March 1 through August 15, 1784* (Vol. 42). Yale University Press.

Gam, S., Guelfi, K. J., & Fournier, P. A. (2016). New insights into enhancing maximal exercise performance through the use of a bitter tastant. *Sports Medicine, 46*, 1385–1390.

Guijarro, C. (2015). A history of the placebo. *Neuroscience History, 2015*(2), 68–80.

Hollister, L. (1960). Placebology: Sense and nonsense. *Current Therapeutic Research, Clinical and Experimental, 2*, 477–483.

Hurst, P., Schipof-Godart, L., Szabo, A., Raglin, J., Hettinga, F., Roelands, B., Lane, A., Foad, A., Coleman, D., & Beedie, C. (2020). The placebo and nocebo effect on sports performance: A systematic review. *European Journal of Sport Science, 20*(3), 279–292.

Kaptchuk, T. J., Kerr, C. E., & Zanger, A. (2009). Placebo controls, exorcisms, and the devil. *The Lancet, 374*(9697), 1234–1235.

Kienle, G. S., & Kiene, H. (1997). The powerful placebo effect: Fact or fiction? *Journal of Clinical Epidemiology, 50*(12), 1311–1318.

Kirsch, I. (1985). Response expectancy as a determinant of experience and behavior. *American Psychologist, 40*(11), 1189.

Kirsch, I. E. (1999). *How expectancies shape experience.* American Psychological Association.

Lindheimer, J., Raglin, J., & Beedie, C. (in press). Placebo Effects in Exercise Outcomes and Sports. In L. Colloca, N. Franklin, & C. Seneviratne (Eds.), *Placebo effects through the lens of translational research.* Oxford University Press.

Loy, B. D., Cameron, M. H., & O'Connor, P. J. (2018). Perceived fatigue and energy are independent unipolar states: Supporting evidence. *Medical Hypotheses, 113*, 46–51.

Meissner, K., Bingel, U., Colloca, L., Wager, T. D., Watson, A., & Flaten, M. A. (2011). The placebo effect: Advances from different methodological approaches. *Journal of Neuroscience, 31*(45), 16117–16124.

Miller, F. G., & Colloca, L. (2009). The legitimacy of placebo treatments in clinical practice: Evidence and ethics. *The American Journal of Bioethics, 9*(12), 39–47.

Peek, C. (1977). A critical look at the theory of placebo. *Biofeedback and Self-regulation, 2*(4), 327–335.

Pierson, W. R. (1961). Amphetamine sulfate and performance: A critique. *JAMA, 177*(5), 345–347.

Pollo, A., Amanzio, M., Arslanian, A., Casadio, C., Maggi, G., & Benedetti, F. (2001). Response expectancies in placebo analgesia and their clinical relevance. *Pain, 93*(1), 77–84.

Quincy, J. (1811). Quincy's Lexicon-medicum. *A New Medical Dictionary.* Longman.

Raglin, J., Szabo, A., Lindheimer, J. B., & Beedie, C. (2020). Understanding placebo and nocebo effects in the context of sport: A psychological perspective. *European Journal of Sport Science, 20*(3), 293–301.

Raglin, J. S. (2007). The psychology of the marathoner: Of one mind and many. *Sports Medicine, 37*, 404–407.

Roberts, A. H. (1995). The powerful placebo revisited: Magnitude of nonspecific effects. *Mind/Body Medicine, 1*(1), 1–10.

Saunders, B., de Oliveira, L. F., da Silva, R. P., de Salles Painelli, V., Gonçalves, L., Yamaguchi, G., Mutti, T., Maciel, E., Roschel, H., & Artioli, G. (2017). Placebo in sports nutrition: A proof-of-principle study involving caffeine supplementation. *Scandinavian Journal of Medicine & Science in Sports, 27*(11), 1240–1247.

Shapiro, A. K. (1968). Semantics of the placebo. *Psychiatric Quarterly, 42*, 653–695.

Smith, G. M., & Beecher, H. K. (1959). Amphetamine sulfate and athletic performance: I. Objective effects. *Journal of the American Medical Association, 170*(5), 542–557.

Smith, G. M., & Beecher, H. K. (1960). Amphetamine, Secobarbital, and Athletic Performance: Ii. Subjective Evaluations of Performances, Mood States, and Physical States. *Journal of the American Medical Association, 172*(14), 1502–1514.

Stewart-Williams, S., & Podd, J. (2004). The placebo effect: Dissolving the expectancy versus conditioning debate. *Psychological Bulletin, 130*(2), 324.

Williamson, J., McColl, R., Mathews, D., Mitchell, J., Raven, P., & Morgan, W. (2001). Hypnotic manipulation of effort sense during dynamic exercise: Cardiovascular responses and brain activation. *Journal of Applied Physiology, 90*(4), 1392–1399.

2

CAN PLACEBO EFFECTS GO WRONG?

The nocebo effect in sport and exercise

Luana Colloca

Introduction

In its broadest sense, the nocebo effect is an unwanted, negative, or unpleasant outcome resulting from the suggestion or belief that a harmful treatment has been received. In early research, nocebo effects were regarded by some as an inconvenient phenomenon that made it harder to test the biological effects of drugs due to participants in the placebo arm of clinical trials experiencing side effects (Manaï et al., 2019). Nevertheless, as research advanced, several authors reported that nocebo effects represent a true experience generated by biological mechanisms (Colloca & Barsky, 2020). The nocebo effect in the context of pain (and other symptoms) includes worsening of existing nociception or pain that is new after a placebo (or negative verbal suggestion) is given. The neurobiology of this involves interactions between multiple changes in brain regions and release of molecules associated with the worsening experience.

While the implications for nocebo effects on sport performance are significant, data are sparse, with most related research focused on the placebo effects generated via positive suggestion and information. However, the largest study to date of placebo and nocebo effects in sport (Hurst et al., 2017), reported a mean nocebo effect across all athletes who received the nocebo treatment, while no equivalent mean placebo effect emerged (i.e., placebo effects were experienced only by a sub-group). Although these data are insufficient to make any generalisable claims as to the relative ubiquity of nocebo and placebo effects in sport, they do support what many athletes, practitioners, and fans know to be the case; negative expectations, beliefs, and emotions in sport can often affect performance in predictably negative ways. For example, most athletes and coaches recognise the idea that the expectation of pain and fatigue

DOI: 10.4324/9781003229001-2

can increase the sensation of pain and fatigue, often resulting in a very real effect negative on performance. The mechanisms of such effects have been extensively researched in clinical pain, which provides clues as to how they might operate in sport.

Nocebo effects in pain

Pain is a complex phenomenon but one that has become a model for the study of placebo and nocebo effects. Nociception refers to the capability to detect painful stimulations that is often studied in the laboratory and it is characterised by physical and/or emotional discomfort (Colloca, 2019). Nocebo hyperalgesia (i.e., heightened sensitivity to pain) refers therefore to increased subjective pain perception after a person receives a placebo treatment or information of potential side effects, negative outcomes, or increased pain (Colloca, 2019). Given that it is widely used in placebo effect research, it is also worth a quick reminder of conditioning, which is an effect generated by the repeated association of a stimulus that elicits a biologically active response, with a cue that does not produce a biologically active response. Repeated association of a stimulus, such as the drug aspirin alongside a cue such as the aspirin pills and box, can eventually lead to a conditioned response such as a reduction in pain, even when the cue is present but the stimulus absent, for example receiving a placebo instead of aspirin. This is known as classical or Pavlovian conditioning, which may occur consciously or subconsciously, meaning that conditioned responses can be generated regardless of whether a person is aware of it.

In order to explore the behavioural and biological mechanisms of nocebo effects in pain, Colloca and Benedetti (2006) used experimental short-lasting phasic stimulations in the form of either electrical shocks or thermal stimulations that can be tailored to the individual levels of detection avoiding harming study participants. In their study, participants were informed about the possibility of receiving a high level of painful (electrical) stimulations, but in fact received either tactile or low-intensity painful stimulations. That is, informing participants about the possibility of receiving high pain caused nociception (i.e., pain to body tissue). These findings indicate that verbal suggestions can induce allodynia (i.e., pain caused by a stimulus that does not normally cause pain) and hyperalgesia (i.e., high pain caused by a stimulus that does not normally cause high pain sensations).

To further understand the differences between conditioning and expectations, Colloca et al. (2008) compared nocebo effects induced by verbal suggestions, as well as those following a high pain conditioning procedure. Results showed that verbal suggestions and the conditioning procedure provoked the same magnitude of nocebo effects with no significant differences. This is counter to most placebo effect research, which suggests that placebo effects induced by expectations are generally lower than those experienced by conditioning procedures (Forsberg et al., 2017; Hurst et al., 2020; Petersen et al., 2014) and highlights the significant contribution expectations and prior experiences can have for inducing nocebo effects.

Colloca et al. (2008) further tested whether there was a causal relation between the number of conditioning trials and the persistence of nocebo effects over time compared to a positive counterpart (i.e., placebo effects). Participants underwent either one or four conditioning sessions with both non-painful and painful stimulations. In the non-painful condition, authors reported that one session of conditioning induced nocebo responses, but not placebo responses. By contrast, both one and four conditioning sessions elicited nocebo effects of similar magnitude independently from the length of conditioning. In a follow-up study, Colagiuri et al. (2015) compared the impact of partial reinforcement on nocebo hyperalgesia using painful electrical shocks in healthy study participants (in psychology, partial reinforcement refers to a behavioural response which is reinforced in only part of the trials and behaviours are often learned slower, but the response tends to be resistant to extinction). Results showed that partial reinforcement elicited nocebo hyperalgesia and the rate of extinction of nocebo hyperalgesia was similar with both the continuous and partial reinforcement. These studies further highlight the ease at which nocebo effects can be induced, and the powerful contribution nocebo effects can have on pain experiences.

Although the above data indicate the sensitivity of inducing nocebo effects, it does not provide an understanding of what may moderate this effect (i.e., when nocebo effects are more likely to occur). A body of evidence has identified what may influence the occurrence of nocebo effects. Some have shown that suggested that such effects may vary across sexes (Shafir et al., 2022), with men being more likely to experience smaller placebo and nocebo effects and prone to experience nocebo effects via verbal suggestions than women. Similarly, people with higher emotional distress, fear of pain and catastrophising (Wang et al., 2022), higher neuroticism and lower detectable threshold (Feldhaus et al., 2021) are likely to experience nocebo effects than their counterparts. Moreover, nocebo effects can generalise within pain-related stimulus modalities (e.g. heat pain, pressure pain) but not to other sensation or symptoms (e.g., itch) (Weng et al., 2022). Experimental research has also shown that nocebo effects can become weaker over time when negative conditioning reinforcement is replaced with positive reinforcement – turning nocebo effects into placebo effects (Meijer et al., 2022) – and social learning can induce negative effects, like increased pain from a placebo treatment (Schenk & Colloca, 2020; Schwartz et al., 2022). This latter finding is especially poignant for team sports where individuals play in teams and compete to win and act together towards an objective. Being in a team where an athlete can see, hear, or directly engage with other athletes experiencing and displaying worsening of performance may increase the likelihood of an athlete experiencing nocebo-like effects (e.g., poor performance) as a result of learning from other athletes.

Nocebo effects across clinical conditions

While the majority of research into nocebo effects is focused on pain, several studies have examined the phenomena across other conditions, such as the motor, respiratory, reproductive, and cardiovascular systems. In particular, motor symptoms such as those associated with Parkinson's disease can be significantly worsened when negative expectations are given. In one study, patients suffering from Parkinson's disease were told that a deep brain stimulation device sending stimulations to the subthalamic region of the brain was turned off, when, in reality, it remained on (Colloca et al., 2004). This information negatively affected bradykinesia (i.e., slowness of motor-control) and those who were openly informed about the (fake) interruption of the deep brain stimulation, experienced a sudden worsening of bradykinesia (Benedetti et al., 2004).

Treatments and post-treatment therapeutic outcomes can be affected by nocebo effects in a paradoxical way. Luparello et al. (1970) demonstrated that asthmatic patients showed widening of the bronchi as a response to bronchoconstrictors when the treatment was described as bronchodilators, and vice versa they showed narrowing of the airways when bronchodilators were presented as bronchoconstrictors. Along these lines, another study demonstrated that healthy participants who thought they were administered a muscle stimulant, experienced muscle tension despite having received a muscle relaxant (Flaten et al., 1999).

Side effects of treatments could also get worse with nocebo effects such as biosimilar treatments and their efficacy (Colloca et al., 2019). For example, in one study (Mondaini et al., 2007), patients with benign enlargement of the prostate gland were given finasteride (5 mg). The treatment was presented as a substance of proven efficacy for the treatment of an enlarged prostate gland. Half of the patients were told that the substance "… may cause erectile dysfunction, decreased libido, problems of ejaculation". The other half were not told about the side effects. Finasteride elicited a 43% rate of sexual side effects in those who were informed about the sexual dysfunction, whereas those to whom the side effects were not told, reported a 15.3% rate of side effects. These studies emphasise how verbal communication that occurs in the daily interaction between patients and clinicians can induce higher occurrence of side effects (Colloca, 2017a, 2017b).

Given that the relief of pain follow surgery is critical, nocebo effects may significantly affect how a patient experiences their pain depending on their expectation of the treatment received. In one study (Colloca et al., 2004) when patients underwent thoracotomy, a surgical procedure to remove lung cancer, in the post-operative window, pain treatments were delivered into the bloodstream through an automated pump, and the timing of the infusion was unknown to the patient. Results showed that when morphine was interrupted openly, anxiety and pain increased significantly whereas when morphine was interrupted surreptitiously, the level of clinical pain remained low. This highlights that participants' awareness of their treatment, and what they believe they have not received may increase anxiety and, in turn, pain.

Nocebo effects in sport and exercise

While most of our understanding of what causes nocebo effects comes from psychology and medicine, there are a handful of studies that have examined this phenomenon on sport and exercise outcomes. In a first study to explicitly investigate nocebo effects on sports performance, Beedie et al. (2007) reported significant decreases in 30-m sprint running speed after the administration of a supplement described as beneficial to endurance performance but harmful to sprint running speed (−1.7%, d = 0.41). The authors also reported significant placebo effects in running speed following the administration of an inert capsule described as beneficial; while no change in mean speed was reported compared to baseline (0.0%, d = 0.0), the authors suggested that the maintenance of speed over six consecutive trials was indicative of a placebo effect. Hurst et al. (2017) investigated the placebo and nocebo effect of a fictitious sport supplement on repeat sprint performance with the inclusion of a no-treatment control group. Compared to no treatment controls, performance decreased when participants received a placebo that was purported to be harmful to performance (−0.9%, d = 0.32), but performance did not change when participants received a placebo that was purported to be beneficial (−0.1%, d = 0.02).

Emadi Andani et al. (2015) investigated the nocebo effect on force production of the right index finger. Compared to no-treatment controls, performance decreased by 12.9% (d = 0.96) following a preconditioning procedure in which the force produced was surreptitiously decreased. Pollo et al. (2012) investigated the nocebo effect of TENS on a leg extension in two separate experiments. In the first experiment, performance was reduced by 11.2% (d = 0.67) when participants believed they had received a harmful treatment. In a second experiment, authors reported a reduction in performance of 8.5% (d = 0.52) after a preconditioning nocebo-inducing procedure.

Colloca et al. (2018) determined the interplay of exercise, placebo, and nocebo effects on pain perception in healthy participants. A challenge when examining exercise performance is that, unlike the contents of a capsule or injection, it is not easy to standardise a dose of exercise across a study. To this aim, the authors developed a machine-controlled isotonic motor task to standardise the exercise task across participants. They used a well-validated model of placebo and nocebo manipulations, reinforcing expectations with a conditioning procedure including visual cues paired with painful stimulations. Participants reported expectations and pain on a trial-by-trial basis. The standardised isotonic exercise task elicited a reduction of pain intensity, and both exercise and placebo induced comparable hypoalgesic effects. When the exercise was added, placebo and nocebo effects were influenced by expectations but were not affected by fatigue or sex. Exercise-, placebo- and nocebo-induced pain modulation are likely to work through distinct mechanisms and neurophysiological research is needed to fully exploit the implications for sport, rehabilitation and pain management (Colloca et al., 2018). In particular, the prospect of optimising patients' expectations and creating intentional conditioned responses within clinical contexts could be exploited placebo effects in medicine (Colloca & Barsky, 2020).

Given the above, Colloca and Barsky (2020) indicated several aspects that could be embedded in daily clinical practice. These recommendations include: 1. Presenting patients with realistic effects of the intervention to avoid violation of expectancies; 2. Favouring positive associations and minimising negative associations between therapeutic interventions and contextual factors; 3. Encouraging patients to communicate their previous or current positive/negative therapeutic experiences; 4. Collecting patients' outcome and treatment expectations as part of the medical history; 5. Aligning patients' expectations with anticipated therapeutic outcome(s); 6. Administering interventions within a positive context (e.g. coping-oriented thoughts) and multisensory cues (e.g. sight, smell, taste stimulation to promote conditioning); and, 7. Framing information about side effects in such a way as to minimise nocebo effects. These (and other aspects) can help patients navigate their expectations of benefits and perceived benefits while enhancing clinical outcomes with optimisation of rehabilitation sessions and pain management protocols.

Biological mechanisms of nocebo effects

Brain imaging techniques have shed light on the neural mechanisms of nocebo effects.

Nocebo can aggravate histaminergic release and itch. In one study, healthy participants experienced itch and higher cooling and histamine concentrations due to an sham "Trans Electrical Nerve Stimulation" (van de Sand et al., 2018). Comparing brain responses during the nocebo manipulation as compared to the control, the authors found an activation of the contralateral rolandic operculum. This part of the brain is associated with the anticipation of a stimulus sensorial sensation and its amplification. In addition, the functional coupling between the insula and the periaqueductal gray was higher during the nocebo condition, suggesting that itch and pain may share similar mechanisms of nocebo-induced facilitation.

In another experiment, study participants underwent dyspnoea because of being exposed to histarinol, an odorous gas, and told that histarinol induces bronchoconstriction (Vlemincx et al., 2021). To induce dyspnoea, a concealed resistive load was inserted into the breathing system. Subsequently, histarinol and a control gas were compared while fMRI data were acquired. The area of the brain named insula paralleled the actual load. By contrast, differences were seen at the level of the periaqueductal gray with higher fMRI signal before the dyspnoea occurred during the anticipation of the worsening of dyspnoea.

Using the open-hidden procedure (Colloca et al., 2004), a pioneering study showed that the effects of strong narcotics such as remifentanil, which is a type of opioid like morphine or fentanyl but with short-acting effect, were reduced by the mere suggestion that the infusion of the drug was stopped. But in reality, the remifentanil was still entering the person's body – they just thought it was being discontinued (Bingel et al., 2011). In this study, the participants who experienced an increase in pain perception after being falsely told the drug had stopped were also evaluated with a technique that measures brain activity called functional magnetic resonance imaging (fMRI). The brain imaging findings suggested that the more a person experienced nocebo-induced pain, the more brain activity there was in a brain structure called the hippocampus which is involved in learning and memory. An extension of this study indicated that the hippocampus bridges nocebo-induced anxiety with an increased responsiveness to nociception (Bingel et al., 2022). Functional connectivity fMRI data has also revealed a correlation between the frontal operculum and hippocampus related to nocebo effects indicating that the affective-cognitive pain pathway and the hippocampus are critically involved during nocebo effects (Kong et al., 2008).

Nocebo effects can be influenced by the order of treatment delivery and associated perception of negative outcomes (Colloca & Benedetti, 2006; Kessner et al., 2013). The therapeutic effect of an ointment is significantly lower when given in the negative than the positive treatment history. Starting a treatment after a treatment perceived as a failure, created nocebo effects paralleled in the brain by a larger activation of the posterior insular cortices, areas connected to nociception and pain amplification (Kessner et al., 2013).

Changes in cortical and subcortical pain-related areas, however, could be a consequence of a facilitation of incoming pain signals at the level of the spinal cord. Büchel and his team were among the first to test this hypothesis (Geuter & Büchel, 2013). An inert cream was applied to the forearm of healthy participants along with a nocebo manipulation (negative conditioning with exposure to high painful stimulations). Participants reported higher pain and at the spinal level, the authors detected a strong activation at the level of the contralateral stimulated dermatomes C5/C6. Thus they provided direct evidence for a mechanism of pain amplification based on nocebo effects occurring before cortical processing of pain signals (Geuter & Büchel, 2013).

Interestingly, the price of a medication given to relieve painful stimulation in a lab can change brain circuitries. Tinnermann and colleagues demonstrated that that labelling an inert treatment as expensive elicited higher nocebo hyperalgesia than labelling it as a less expensive treatment (Tinnermann et al., 2017). The price affected the neural signalling in brain regions such as cortex, brainstem, and spinal cord. Brain activity localised in the prefrontal cortex accounted for the impact of the price on nocebo effects. In addition, price affected the functional coupling (aka the extent to which parts of the brain communicate) among areas such as prefrontal areas, brainstem, and spinal cord. Thus, nocebo effects can tune the brain activity underlying modulation of pain processing (Tinnermann et al., 2017).

At the molecular level, nocebo effects in the pain arena have been primarily linked to the release of a hormone called cholecystokinin (CCK), which increases during times of heightened anxiety and panic (Benedetti et al., 1997; Benedetti et al., 2006). A study showed that verbal suggestions of increased pain induced an activation of adrenocorticotropic hormone and cortisol plasma concentrations along with perceived pain sensation after a tourniquet. Proglumide binds type-A/B receptors of CCK and, when given before the nocebo suggestions, blocked nocebo hyperalgesia, indicating an involvement of CCK in the hyperalgesic effects (Benedetti et al., 2006). In general, research points to a relationship between nocebo effects and how anxiety and stress are regulated. Other hormones play a role in nocebo (i.e., release of cortisol) contributing to nocebo-induced worsening of pain and other symptoms. Moreover, rate and magnitude of nocebo effects have been associated with maternal plasma cortisol levels during the three trimesters of pregnancy. Participants who showed 4 adverse events in adulthood during a nocebo challenge had prenatal maternal cortisol above normal levels (Benedetti et al., 2022).

Implications and future directions

Nocebo effect research has tangible implications for those in sport and exercise. First, nocebo effects are the result of neurobiological mechanisms and a cascade of neuropeptides released in the brain. Sport-related performance is damped by a nocebo effect (Colloca et al., 2018; Hurst et al., 2020). Studies illustrating how beliefs of medical professionals that are expressed via subtle cues and behaviours, can influence patient expectations and outcomes (Gracely et al., 1985) and are easily translated into the sport and exercise context.

But by comparison with domains such as psychology and medicine, research into nocebo effects on sport and exercise is severely lacking. This paucity of evidence in relation to nocebo effects in sports performance is somewhat surprising given that, theoretically, negative information or beliefs about a legitimate treatment could offset some or all of the beneficial effects of that treatment. While it is unlikely that an athlete would use a treatment they believed was harmful to their performance, it does highlight that if an athlete does not fully believe in a treatment, they may not fully benefit from it. This is perhaps not only true of an athlete using, for example, an ergogenic aid, but also an exerciser using exercise as an intervention in health, where negative expectations of pain or fatigue might elicit nocebo effects that result in the cessation of the exercise and are thereby counterproductive health outcomes for the person.

The decrease in performances shown by Beedie et al. (2007) and Hurst et al. (2017) highlight the significant implications nocebo effects can have for athlete's performance and future research is needed to identify what may increase the likelihood of an athlete experiencing a nocebo effect. Identifying those who respond negatively to a placebo is important for both clinical and applied practice.

As reported above, nocebo effects may be easier to induce than placebo effects (Colloca et al., 2008; Hurst et al., 2017). Providing a clear explanation for this is difficult but, as reported by others (Baumeister et al., 2001), negative information can have a stronger influence on behaviour than positive information. Rozin and Royzman (2001) reported that "in most situations, negative events are more salient, potent, dominant in combinations, and generally efficacious than positive events" (p. 297). People are more likely to react to negative information more pertinently than to positive information (Colloca & Barsky, 2020). Given this, when an athlete or exerciser is given both negative and positive information about a treatment, they may be more cognisant and process the negative information more consciously than the positive information. As a result, athletes and exercisers may therefore have greater negative expectations of the treatment and as a result be more likely to experience pain, fatigue, and reductions in performance. These results further underscore the importance of those working in sport and exercise to be aware of how they communicate with their athletes during administration of treatments (see also Andy Lane's chapter).

Acknowledgements

The author has received funding by the National Institute of Dental Craniofacial Research (NIDCR R01DE025946, PI Colloca), the National Center for Complementary and Integrative Health (NCCIH R01AT01033 & R01 AT011347-01A1 PI: Colloca).

References

Baumeister, R. F., Bratslavsky, E., Finkenauer, C., & Vohs, K. D. (2001). Bad is stronger than good. *Review of General Psychology, 5*(4), 323–370.

Beedie, C. J., Coleman, D. A., & Foad, A. J. (2007). Positive and negative placebo effects resulting from the deceptive administration of an ergogenic aid. *International Journal of Sport Nutrition and Exercise Metabolism, 17*(3), 259–269.

Benedetti, F., Amanzio, M., Casadio, C., Oliaro, A., & Maggi, G. (1997). Blockade of nocebo hyperalgesia by the cholecystokinin antagonist proglumide. *Pain, 71*(2), 135–140.

Benedetti, F., Amanzio, M., Fabio, G., Karen, C.-B., Claudia, A., & Aziz, S. (2022). Are nocebo effects in adulthood linked to prenatal maternal cortisol levels? *Clinical Neuropsychiatry, 19*(5), 298–306.

Benedetti, F., Amanzio, M., Vighetti, S., & Asteggiano, G. (2006). The biochemical and neuroendocrine bases of the hyperalgesic nocebo effect. *Journal of Neuroscience, 26*(46), 12014–12022.

Benedetti, F., Colloca, L., Lanotte, M., Bergamasco, B., Torre, E., & Lopiano, L. (2004). Autonomic and emotional responses to open and hidden stimulations of the human subthalamic region. *Brain Research Bulletin, 63*(3), 203–211.

Bingel, U., Wanigasekera, V., Wiech, K., Ni Mhuircheartaigh, R., Lee, M. C., Ploner, M., & Tracey, I. (2011). The effect of treatment expectation on drug efficacy: Imaging the analgesic benefit of the opioid remifentanil. *Science Translational Medicine, 3*(70), 70ra14.

Bingel, U., Wiech, K., Ritter, C., Wanigasekera, V., Ní Mhuircheartaigh, R., Lee, M. C., Ploner, M., & Tracey, I. (2022). Hippocampus mediates nocebo impairment of opioid analgesia through changes in functional connectivity. *European Journal of Neuroscience, 56*(2), 3967–3978.

Colagiuri, B., Quinn, V. F., & Colloca, L. (2015). Nocebo hyperalgesia, partial reinforcement, and extinction. *The Journal of Pain, 16*(10), 995–1004.

Colloca, L. (2017a). Nocebo effects can make you feel pain. *Science, 358*(6359), 44.

Colloca, L. (2017b). Tell me the truth and I will not be harmed: Informed consents and nocebo effects. *The American Journal of Bioethics, 17*(6), 46–48.

Colloca, L. (2019). The placebo effect in pain therapies. *Annual Review of Pharmacology and Toxicology, 59*, 191–211.

Colloca, L., & Barsky, A. J. (2020). Placebo and nocebo effects. *New England Journal of Medicine, 382*(6), 554–561.

Colloca, L., & Benedetti, F. (2006). How prior experience shapes placebo analgesia. *Pain, 124*(1–2), 126–133.

Colloca, L., Corsi, N., & Fiorio, M. (2018). The interplay of exercise, placebo and nocebo effects on experimental pain. *Scientific Reports, 8*(1), 1–11.

Colloca, L., Lopiano, L., Lanotte, M., & Benedetti, F. (2004). Overt versus covert treatment for pain, anxiety, and Parkinson's disease. *The Lancet Neurology, 3*(11), 679–684.

Colloca, L., Panaccione, R., & Murphy, T. K. (2019). The clinical implications of nocebo effects for biosimilar therapy. *Frontiers in Pharmacology, 10*, 1372.

Colloca, L., Sigaudo, M., & Benedetti, F. (2008). The role of learning in nocebo and placebo effects. *Pain, 136*(1–2), 211–218.

Emadi Andani, M., Tinazzi, M., Corsi, N., & Fiorio, M. (2015). Modulation of inhibitory corticospinal circuits induced by a nocebo procedure in motor performance. *PLoS One, 10*(4), e0125223.

Feldhaus, M. H., Horing, B., Sprenger, C., & Büchel, C. (2021). Association of nocebo hyperalgesia and basic somatosensory characteristics in a large cohort. *Scientific Reports, 11*(1), 1–12.

Flaten, M. A., Simonsen, T., & Olsen, H. (1999). Drug-related information generates placebo and nocebo responses that modify the drug response. *Psychosomatic Medicine, 61*(2), 250–255.

Forsberg, J. T., Martinussen, M., & Flaten, M. A. (2017). The placebo analgesic effect in healthy individuals and patients: A meta-analysis. *Psychosomatic Medicine, 79*(4), 388–394.

Geuter, S., & Büchel, C. (2013). Facilitation of pain in the human spinal cord by nocebo treatment. *Journal of Neuroscience, 33*(34), 13784–13790.

Gracely, R., Dubner, R., Deeter, W., & Wolskee, P. (1985). Clinicians' expectations influence placebo analgesia. *Lancet, 43*(8419), 43.

Hurst, P., Foad, A., Coleman, D., & Beedie, C. (2017). Athletes intending to use sports supplements are more likely to respond to a placebo. *Medicine & Science in Sports & Exercise,* 49(9), 1877–1883.

Hurst, P., Schipof-Godart, L., Szabo, A., Raglin, J., Hettinga, F., Roelands, B., Lane, A., Foad, A., Coleman, D., & Beedie, C. (2020). The placebo and nocebo effect on sports performance: A systematic review. *European Journal of Sport Science, 20*(3), 279–292.

Kessner, S., Wiech, K., Forkmann, K., Ploner, M., & Bingel, U. (2013). The effect of treatment history on therapeutic outcome: An experimental approach. *JAMA Internal Medicine, 173*(15), 1468–1469.

Kong, J., Gollub, R. L., Polich, G., Kirsch, I., LaViolette, P., Vangel, M., Rosen, B., & Kaptchuk, T. J. (2008). A functional magnetic resonance imaging study on the neural mechanisms of hyperalgesic nocebo effect. *Journal of Neuroscience, 28*(49), 13354–13362.

Luparello, T. J., Leist, N., Lourie, C. H., & Sweet, P. (1970). The interaction of psychologic stimuli and pharmacologic agents on airway reactivity in asthmatic subjects. *Psychosomatic Medicine, 32*(5), 509–514.

Manaï, M., van Middendorp, H., Veldhuijzen, D. S., Huizinga, T. W., & Evers, A. W. (2019). How to prevent, minimize, or extinguish nocebo effects in pain: A narrative review on mechanisms, predictors, and interventions. *Pain Reports, 4*(3), e699.

Meijer, S., Van Middendorp, H., Peerdeman, K. J., & Evers, A. W. (2022). Counterconditioning as treatment to reduce nocebo effects in persistent physical symptoms: Treatment protocol and study design. *Frontiers in Psychology, 13,* 806409.

Mondaini, N., Gontero, P., Giubilei, G., Lombardi, G., Cai, T., Gavazzi, A., & Bartoletti, R. (2007). Finasteride 5 mg and sexual side effects: How many of these are related to a nocebo phenomenon? *The Journal of Sexual Medicine, 4*(6), 1708–1712.

Petersen, G. L., Finnerup, N. B., Colloca, L., Amanzio, M., Price, D. D., Jensen, T. S., & Vase, L. (2014). The magnitude of nocebo effects in pain: A meta-analysis. *Pain®, 155*(8), 1426–1434.

Pollo, A., Carlino, E., Vase, L., & Benedetti, F. (2012). Preventing motor training through nocebo suggestions. *European Journal of Applied Physiology, 112,* 3893–3903.

Rozin, P., & Royzman, E. B. (2001). Negativity bias, negativity dominance, and contagion. *Personality and Social Psychology Review, 5*(4), 296–320.

Schenk, L. A., & Colloca, L. (2020). The neural processes of acquiring placebo effects through observation. *Neuroimage, 209,* 116510.

Schwartz, M., Fischer, L.-M., Bläute, C., Stork, J., Colloca, L., Zöllner, C., & Klinger, R. (2022). Observing treatment outcomes in other patients can elicit augmented placebo effects on pain treatment: A double-blinded randomized clinical trial with patients with chronic low back pain. *Pain, 163*(7), 1313.

Shafir, R., Olson, E., & Colloca, L. (2022). The neglect of sex: A call to action for including sex as a biological variable in placebo and nocebo research. *Contemporary Clinical Trials*, 106734.

Tinnermann, A., Geuter, S., Sprenger, C., Finsterbusch, J., & Büchel, C. (2017). Interactions between brain and spinal cord mediate value effects in nocebo hyperalgesia. *Science*, *358*(6359), 105–108.

van de Sand, M. F., Menz, M. M., Sprenger, C., & Büchel, C. (2018). Nocebo-induced modulation of cerebral itch processing–an fMRI study. *Neuroimage*, *166*, 209–218.

Vlemincx, E., Sprenger, C., & Büchel, C. (2021). Expectation and dyspnoea: The neurobiological basis of respiratory nocebo effects. *European Respiratory Journal*, 58(3), 2003008.

Wang, Y., Chan, E., Dorsey, S. G., Campbell, C. M., & Colloca, L. (2022). Who are the placebo responders? A cross-sectional cohort study for psychological determinants. *Pain*, *163*(6), 1078–1090.

Weng, L., Peerdeman, K. J., Della Porta, D., van Laarhoven, A. I., & Evers, A. W. (2022). Can placebo and nocebo effects generalize within pain modalities and across somatosensory sensations? *Pain*, *163*(3), 548–559.

3

CAN A PLACEBO EFFECT MAKE ME FASTER?

Evidence for placebo effects as performance enhancers in sport

Guilherme Matta, Florentina Hettinga, and Andrew Edwards

Introduction

In the past two decades, research has demonstrated that placebo effects can significantly influence athletes' performance. A systematic review of 32 experimental studies involving over 1500 participants (Hurst et al., 2020) reported small to moderate placebo effects associated with the hidden administration of nutritional (e.g., caffeine, sodium bicarbonate, carbohydrates) and mechanical ergogenic aids (e.g., transcutaneous electrical nerve stimulation, kinesiology tape, ischemic preconditioning). Given that marginal differences in performance can determine differences between winners and losers (Hopkins et al., 1999), the effects reported are potentially meaningful in real-world competitive settings. To provide the reader with an understanding of its potential impact in sport, the aim of this chapter is to provide a brief summary of the studies investigating placebo effects across different treatments on various types of sport performance outcomes.

Types of placebos

Various methods by which to induce placebo effects have been reported in the sport and exercise science literature (Beedie & Foad, 2009; Hurst et al., 2020), the most prevalent being in studies of purported nutritional or pharmacological ergogenic aids (e.g., caffeine, sodium bicarbonate and anabolic steroids; Hurst et al., 2020). This is understandable given that manipulating participant expectations about what they have received is far easier to do with a nutritional and pharmacological aid (Best et al., 2018; Gurton et al., 2022) than is the case with other treatments, for example exercise (Lindheimer et al., 2020;

DOI: 10.4324/9781003229001-3

readers are directed to Chapter 9 of this book for a more in-depth discussion). That being said, there are a handful of studies that have attempted to manipulate participants' expectations about what they received in relation to arguably more elaborate ergogenic aids, such as transcutaneous electrical nerve stimulation (TENS), ischemic preconditioning and tennis rackets (Ferreira et al., 2016; Rossettini et al., 2018). Below, we outline some of the studies that have examined different types of placebos and their impact on sport performance.

In relation to nutritional or pharmacological ergogenic aids, Hurst et al. (2020) reported that placebo effects induced by a purported prohibited substance had the largest effects on performance. That is, placebo effects of sham anabolic steroids and of sham recombinant human erythropoietin were much larger (effect size range = 0.72 to 2.15) than for sham caffeine (effect size range = –0.08 to 0.88) or sham sodium bicarbonate (effect size = 0.13). For instance, Ross et al. (2015) reported significant improvements in running performance when participants self-administered subcutaneous saline injections (i.e., a placebo), believing it to be "OxyRBX", a substance with similar effects to recombinant human erythropoietin (EPO). The participants reported reductions in physical effort, increased motivation, and improved recovery following administration of the placebo injections. Similarly, Maganaris et al. (2000) reported improvements of 3.5, 4.2 and 5.2%, for bench press, deadlift and squat, respectively, when participants received a placebo but were informed it was a potent anabolic steroid.

Hurst et al. (2020) also provided an overview of 12 studies that investigated placebo effects induced by mechanical ergogenic aids. These involved TENS, magnetic wristbands, cold-water immersion, ischemic preconditioning, and kinesiology tape. Hurst et al. reported moderate to large effects induced by TENS with improvements in performance of up to 14.4% (although it must be stressed that these larger effects were reported on more finer motor control movements of the finger; Rossettini et al., 2018). Placebo effects induced by ischemic preconditioning were also investigated, with Marocolo et al. (2015) reporting an improvement of 0.9% in swimming performance when the placebo was administered in comparison to controls. However, Ferreira et al. (2016) failed to find any significant differences between the placebo and control (0.1% change), although they found significant improvements after ischemic preconditioning (1.2%). Broatch et al. (2014) investigated the physiological responses to cold-water immersion compared to placebo, reporting that the placebo was superior to controls in the recovery of muscle strength. Further, one study investigated the effects of magnetic wristbands, which were presented as likely to improve balance, strength and flexibility (Brazier et al., 2014) but failed to find any differences in performance over different tests.

A few studies have examined placebo effects induced by sports equipment on performance. Guillot et al. (2012) analysed how a modified tennis racket, purported to enhance performance, affected tennis serve accuracy scores. They found that 'placebo rackets' enhanced accuracy of performance by 5.7%, in comparison to controls. In another study, Blumenstein et al. (2021) investigated whether hypothetical differences in rolling-ski resistance affected junior cross-country skiers' performance over a time-trial. Although the rolling resistance was kept constant, participants' performance decreased when they believed the roller skis had higher resistance; thus, their mistaken belief was that this would impede performance (i.e., a nocebo effect; see Colloca's chapter for more details, Chapter 2). The combined results of both studies suggest that athletes' beliefs and perceptions about their equipment may also affect their performance.

Collectively, the above evidence indicates that placebo effects can significantly improve sport performance across a variety of different treatments and interventions. Given that athletes often search for small margins to improve performance (<1%; Hopkins et al., 1999), the results of the studies reported above highlight the contribution placebo effects could potentially make to an athlete's performance. In addition, what this evidence highlights is that placebo effects may be larger for some ergogenic aids (e.g., prohibited substances and TENS) than others (e.g., magnetic wristbands and kinesiotape) and that they may be more impactful in discrete/fine skills (e.g., Rossettini et al., 2018) than whole-body/gross movements (e.g., Ross et al., 2015; Chapter 10). An athlete's expectations or prior experience of using an ergogenic aid is likely to play a significant role in how effective it may be in terms of their performance. Findings related to mechanical placebos are particularly interesting given recent men's and women's world records in long-distance running have been broken by athletes wearing running shoes that are purported to increase performance by ~4%. It is likely that the new shoes, which are composed of a full-length carbon-fibre plate embedded within the shoes' foam, deliver a mechanical advantage (Hunter et al., 2019), but potential placebo effects cannot be disregarded until full placebo-controlled trials are published.

Placebo effects and exercise demands

Above we illustrated the different ways of inducing placebo effects reported in the sports science research literature. To understand how placebo effects may vary depending on sport type, in the sections below the results of studies examining placebo effects induced by purported ergogenic aids on endurance, sprint, and muscle strength performance are summarised. Further, we also address the body of literature which has examined how placebo-like effects can be induced by the manipulation of information the athlete receives about their opponent.

Endurance performance

One of the most common methods in which to examine placebo effects on sport performance has been during endurance-based tasks. In one of the first placebo effect studies to examine placebo effects on sport, Clark et al. (2000) examined the effect of carbohydrate supplementation, which is widely used in sport, during 40-km cycling time-trials. Clark et al. (2000) gave 43 endurance cyclists a drink containing either carbohydrates or a placebo and found that when participants received a placebo described as carbohydrate, performance increased by 4.3%. In a similar study, however, Hulston and Jeukendrup (2009) did not find any placebo effect during an endurance-based cycling time-trial after participants received a placebo described as carbohydrate. Unfortunately, authors did not examine what may have caused, or not caused, placebo effects in both studies, and it is uncertain as to why differences emerged. Importantly, however, what it does highlight is that placebo effects may not always be induced.

Caffeine, like carbohydrate, is widely used by athletes. Unlike carbohydrate solution however, it is relatively easy to 'disguise' as a placebo, and this factor, combined with its strong evidence base (Grgic et al., 2020), makes it an ideal vehicle to for placebo effects research. As a result, several studies have examined placebo effects of caffeine on sport performance outcomes. In the first study to examine placebo effects of caffeine, Beedie et al. (2006) reported a mean of 1.4% and 3.1% placebo effect on power output over 10-km cycling time-trials when participants believed they had ingested a capsule containing 4.5 mg.kg^{-1} and 0.9 mg.kg^{-1} of caffeine, respectively. The same authors also showed that the performance of participants decreased by −1.4% when they correctly believed that they had ingested a placebo. Similarly, Pires et al. (2018) found that caffeine, and placebo perceived as caffeine, improved peak power output by 11.2% and 11.9%, and time to exhaustion by 15.4% and 17.4%, respectively, and Hurst et al. (2019) reported that when athletes believed they had received caffeine, their time to run 1000-m improved to the same magnitude as when they had actually received caffeine (1.9% versus 1.8%, respectively).

Although the above studies reported a mean placebo effect of caffeine on sport performance, Foad et al. (2008) found no differences in 40-km cycling time-trials when participants believed they had ingested caffeine but received a placebo (0.1%). Authors conducted follow-up interviews with participants after the completion of the study (Beedie et al., 2008) and reported that 5 of the 14 participants in the study reported a placebo effect, which was associated with an increase in psychological (e.g., motivation, pain tolerance and fatigue resilience) and physiological (e.g., increase in oxygen uptake and blood lactate) processes. Whereas for the 9 participants that reported no placebo effects, authors found that participants failed to experience changes in psychology or physiology, suggesting a subtle interplay between bottom-up and top-down regulation that may influence whether an athlete responds to a placebo. That is, after receiving a placebo, an athlete may consciously search for clues that the substance will take effect, either through an increase in arousal or heart rate, and, in turn, influence their likelihood of experiencing a placebo effect. This finding is partially supported by Saunders et al. (2017), who reported that participants who incorrectly identified caffeine after they received placebo, were more likely to show a placebo effect than those who correctly identified a placebo. This highlights the cognitive processes that athletes may consider during an experimental trial and how this may interact with the administration of the treatment in question, and in turn, influence performance outcomes.

Other studies to examine placebo effects during endurance performance have examined the administration of sodium bicarbonate, beta-alanine and anabolic steroids. McClung and Collins (2007) reported that when runners ingested sodium bicarbonate or a placebo described as sodium bicarbonate before a 1000-m time-trial, performance was improved by 1.7% and 1.5%, respectively. However, when participants received sodium bicarbonate expecting a placebo, performance changed by −0.3%, suggesting that benefits associated with sodium bicarbonate ingestion are at least in part based on the expectancy of receiving an ergogenic aid. Bellinger and Minahan (2016) also reported improvements in performance during 1-km cycling time-trials following the overt (2.4%) and hidden (1.8%) administration of beta-alanine, although the differences were not significant.

In summary, several studies have confirmed that placebo effects of nutritional and pharmacological ergogenic aids can improve endurance performance. These data have identified that when an athlete is given a placebo, but expects an ergogenic aid, this can significantly improve their ability to perform over an endurance-based task. However, it must be stressed that not all studies reported a mean placebo effect, and it is likely that, by its nature, longer events increase the opportunity for athletes to consciously search for evidence that what they expected to have received is having an effect, either psychologically or physiologically. If this is not apparent, then placebo effects may be less likely to be induced.

Sprint performance

In the majority of sporting events (e.g., basketball, football, Rugby), the ability for an athlete to sprint quickly and repeatedly is a key attribute in sport. More importantly, the majority of sprinting in these events occurs over relatively short distances of less than 40m (<40 m; Cross et al., 2015) and are of short durations of less than 4 seconds (<4 seconds; Spencer et al., 2005). Understanding if placebo effects can influence sprint performance has therefore been used an outcome measure in a number of studies (Hurst et al., 2020). In the first study to examine placebo effects on sprinting, Beedie et al. (2007) analysed whether a placebo capsule improved and/or worsened speed achieved during 3 × 30-m repeated sprints. Athletes (N = 42) were randomised to two groups, with the group receiving negative information (i.e., capsule will worsen performance), experiencing a mean −1.7% drop in speed, while the positive information group (i.e., capsule will improve performance) maintaining a higher speed throughout the repeated sprints. These results showed that when athletes received positive information about a placebo, they ran faster over successive trials that when they received negative information.

In a further study investigating placebo effects on sprinting performance, Tolusso et al. (2015) investigated whether a placebo drink described as an ergogenic substance affected performance during 3 x running-based anaerobic sprint tests (RAST) completed over two consecutive days. They reported improved peak and mean power output when compared to the control condition. Similarly, de la Vega et al. (2017) investigated whether a fictitious and inert drink affected 200-m sprint performance. Their participants were split into three groups that only differed in the information received: 1) positive group: the drink improves performance; 2) partial positive: the drink may or may not improve performance; 3) neutral: the drink does not affect performance. They found that the positive group improved performance by 6.2% compared to the baseline trial, whereas partial positive and neutral were not significantly different to baseline.

While the above studies highlight that expectations of a placebo treatment described as a supplement can improve or worsen performance, the designs used were limited by the non-inclusion of a no-treatment control group. No-treatment control groups are important to help delineate whether any changes are a result of placebo effects and not placebo responses (such as regression to the mean; see Chapter 1 for more detail). In short, to ensure changes observed in the placebo treatment are in fact due to the psychosocial environment surrounding the administration of treatment and not non-specific factors associated with methodological and/or statistical artefacts, research needs to include a no-treatment control in their study design. Given this, Hurst et al. (2017) replicated the study by Beedie et al. (2007) and examined placebo and nocebo effects induced by an inert capsule described either as a potent supplement that would improve or decrease sprinting performance, and compared this to a no-treatment control. Results showed that compared to controls, speed significantly reduced when participants received the capsule purported to worsen performance (−0.9%). However, in the positive-information group, mean performance was no different to controls. Thus, while a nocebo effect was observed, no mean placebo effect emerged. This highlights the importance for research to include no-treatment groups to ensure inferences about a placebo (or nocebo) effect are reliable.

Strength performance

Another fundamental physical attribute in sport is strength. As a result, several studies have examined what impact placebo effects can have on the amount of weight a person can lift. The first study to do so, Ariel and Saville (1972), administered a placebo pill described as an anabolic steroid for four weeks, and reported that force production improved by an average of 9.5% compared to baseline. It was not until the turn of the century, however, that another study examined the placebo effect on strength outcomes. Maganaris et al. (2000) administered a placebo described as a powerful anabolic steroid and, like Ariel and Saville (1972), participants improved the amount of weight they could lift by on average 4.6%. Authors provided further insight into the impact expectations about placebos can have on strength and reported that when a subgroup of athletes were informed that they had received a placebo mid-trial, performance improvements dissipated, where they remained in the other subgroup, who were told it was a potent substance. These results highlight the significant role expectations have for inducing placebo effects.

Kalasountas et al. (2007) adopted a similar design to Maganaris et al. (2000) and informed their participants that they would receive a "strong combination of amino acids" and that effects on strength performance would be immediate. They reported an average improvement of 11% in performance and, when the true nature of the substance was disclosed, like Maganaris et al. (2000), force production returned to baseline. Pollo et al. (2008) investigated the effects of a placebo drink, described as containing a high dose of caffeine on leg extension performance. In the first part of the experiment, they found a significant increase in muscle work (11.8%) when participants received a placebo. Subsequently, they used a conditioning procedure whereby the administration of the placebo drink was coupled with a surreptitious reduction in the amount of weight lifted, to enforce beliefs that the task was easier after taking the drink. They reported an even larger improvement of 22.1% in muscle work when the load was restored to baseline. Similarly, Duncan et al. (2009) investigated the effects of a placebo perceived as caffeine on leg extension performance. When participants perceived they ingested caffeine before the task, they completed more repetitions (at 60% of 1RM) and increased the total weight lifted with lower ratings of perceived exertion. Collectively, the results of this study suggest robust placebo effects induced by different interventions on strength performance and that conditioning protocols might induce even larger placebo effects.

Competitive performance

Given that placebo effects are induced by social interactions, studies have investigated how the presence of opponents might alter athletes' expectations about the exercise task and induce placebo effects. Several studies report performance improvements when cyclists compete against an on-screen avatar compared to individual time-trials, which have been related to changes in psychological outputs, such as motivation, attentional focus and fatigue tolerance (Davies et al., 2016; Jones et al., 2013; Williams et al., 2015). Recently, several studies analysed how interactions with virtual opponents affect performance in a laboratory-controlled environment. Stone et al. (2012) reported a mean improvement in performance of 1.7% during a 4,000-m cycling time-trial when participants competed against an avatar riding at 2% higher power output than their baseline. Similarly, Corbett et al. (2012) found performance improvements when participants competed against an avatar representing their best baseline performance and Williams et al. (2015) reported improvements of 2.8% during 16-km cycling time-trial performance when participants competed against their own best individual time-trial performance, believed to be an opponent of similar performance capacity. Williams et al. (2015) also reported reduced internal attentional focus during the competition trial and increased motivation, which resulted in increased fatigue tolerance. Konings and Hettinga (2018) showed that 4-km cycling time-trial performance improved when participants competed against a virtual avatar representing their baseline performance, in comparison to riding alone. They reported that improvements were accompanied by a greater decline in muscle force over the duration and changes in pacing, mainly at the start and end of the time-trials, although ratings of perceived exertion were the same. Finally, Ansdell (2018) found improvements in 4-km cycling time-trial performance when athletes competed against an on-screen avatar surreptitiously riding at 2% higher power outputs than a baseline trial. However, performance improvements were not accompanied by greater peripheral fatigue, attributing these changes to an altered pacing strategy.

Collectively, the results of these studies show robust improvements in performance when athletes compete against a virtual opponent, irrespective of the intervention adopted. The mechanisms behind such improvements can be associated to alterations in psychophysiological factors, such as muscle force decline, greater anaerobic energy contribution, increased motivation, willingness to sustain fatigue, and changes in pacing.

Conclusions

Evidence suggests that a competitive edge can be obtained through augmenting expectations in the effectiveness of performance-enhancing substances, such as caffeine, sodium bicarbonate and anabolic steroids, as well as about who the athlete competes against. The abundance of studies examining placebo effects on sport have established that all types of treatments used by athletes are likely to be influenced by the placebo effect. Further, placebos are likely to augment performance across several sporting outcomes, such as endurance, sprinting and strength, and might provide an athlete a significant edge to their performance. It is plausible to suggest, therefore, that most interventions adopted in sports sciences, whether through nutritional or mechanical ergogenic aids, equipment manipulation, or the presence of competitors, might have at least some placebo components and, given that the difference between first and last place can be extremely small in elite sport, such competitive advantages are likely to be meaningful to athletes. It should be recognised, however, that most studies presented here were conducted in highly controlled laboratory environments, which makes the extrapolation of the results to real-world settings difficult. A need exists to identify the degree to which placebo effects occur during intense competition, where pressure, anxiety and nerves are likely to be far higher, and which might as a result dampen, or potentially enhance, the performance impact of a placebo effect. It is important that future studies consider the effects of participants' expectations and prior experiences on different interventions, attempting to control for changes in performance induced by placebo effects and how these operate within real-world environments.

References

Ansdell, P. (2018). Deception improves time trial erformance in well-trained cyclists without augmented fatigue. *Medicine & Science in Sports & Exercise*, *50*(4), 809–816. https://doi.org/10.1249/MSS.0000000000001483

Ariel, G., & Saville, W. (1972). Effect of anabolic steroids on reflex components. *Journal of Applied Physiology*, *32*(6), 795–797.

Beedie, C. J., Coleman, D. A., & Foad, A. J. (2007). Positive and negative placebo effects resulting from the deceptive administration of an ergogenic aid. *International Journal of Sport Nutrition and Exercise Metabolism*, *17*(3), 259–269.

Beedie, C. J., & Foad, A. J. (2009). The placebo effect in sports performance: A brief review. *Sports Medicine*, *39*, 313–329.

Beedie, C. J., Foad, A. J., & Coleman, D. A. (2008). Identification of placebo responsive participants in 40km laboratory cycling performance. *Journal of Sports Science & Medicine*, *7*(1), 166.

Beedie, C. J., Stuart, E. M., Coleman, D. A., & Foad, A. J. (2006). Placebo effects of caffeine on cycling performance. *Medicine and Science in Sports and Exercise*, *38*(12), 2159.

Bellinger, P. M., & Minahan, C. L. (2016). The effect of β-alanine supplementation on cycling time trials of different length. *European Journal of Sport Science*, *16*(7), 829–836.

Best, R., Spears, I. R., Hurst, P., & Berger, N. J. (2018). The development of a menthol solution for use during sport and exercise. *Beverages*, *4*(2), 44.

Blumenstein, B., Abrahamsen, F. E., & Losnegard, T. (2021). Placebo and nocebo in sports: Potential effects of hypothetical differences in roll resistance on roller ski performance. *Translational Sports Medicine*, *4*(3), 401–408.

Brazier, J., Sinclair, J., & Bottoms, L. (2014). The effects of hologram wristbands and placebo on athletic performance. *Kinesiology*, *46*(1), 109–116.

Broatch, J. R., Petersen, A., & Bishop, D. J. (2014). Postexercise cold water immersion benefits are not greater than the placebo effect. *Medicine & Science in Sports & Exercise*, 46(11), 2139–2147.

Clark, V. R., Hopkins, W. G., Hawley, J. A., & Burke, L. M. (2000). Placebo effect of carbohydrate feedings during a 40-km cycling time trial. *Medicine and science in sports and exercise*, 32(9), 1642–1647.

Corbett, J., Barwood, M. J., Ouzounoglou, A., Thelwell, R., & Dicks, M. (2012). Influence of competition on performance and pacing during cycling exercise. *Medicine & Science in Sports & Exercise*, 44(3), 509–515.

Cross, M. R., Brughelli, M., Brown, S. R., Samozino, P., Gill, N. D., Cronin, J. B., & Morin, J.-B. (2015). Mechanical properties of sprinting in elite rugby union and rugby league. *International Journal of Sports Physiology and Performance*, 10(6), 695–702.

Davies, M. J., Clark, B., Welvaert, M., Skorski, S., Garvican-Lewis, L. A., Saunders, P., & Thompson, K. G. (2016). Effect of environmental and feedback interventions on pacing profiles in cycling: A meta-analysis. *Frontiers in Physiology*, 7, 591.

de la Vega, R., Alberti, S., Ruíz-Barquín, R., Soós, I., & Szabo, A. (2017). Induced beliefs about a fictive energy drink influences 200-m sprint performance. *European journal of sport science*, 17(8), 1084–1089.

Duncan, M. J., Lyons, M., & Hankey, J. (2009). Placebo effects of caffeine on short-term resistance exercise to failure. *International Journal of Sports Physiology and Performance*, 4(2), 244–253.

Ferreira, T. N., Sabino-Carvalho, J. L., Lopes, T. R., Ribeiro, I. C., Succi, J. E., Da Silva, A. C., & Silva, B. M. (2016). Ischemic preconditioning and repeated sprint swimming: A placebo and nocebo study. *Medicine & Science in Sports & Exercise*, 48(10), 1967–1975.

Foad, A. J., Beedie, C. J., & Coleman, D. A. (2008). Pharmacological and psychological effects of caffeine ingestion in 40-km cycling performance. *Medicine and Science in Sports and Exercise*, 40(1), 158.

Grgic, J., Grgic, I., Pickering, C., Schoenfeld, B. J., Bishop, D. J., & Pedisic, Z. (2020). Wake up and smell the coffee: Caffeine supplementation and exercise performance—an umbrella review of 21 published meta-analyses. *British Journal of Sports Medicine*, 54(11), 681–688.

Guillot, A., Genevois, C., Desliens, S., Saieb, S., & Rogowski, I. (2012). Motor imagery and 'placebo-racket effects' in tennis serve performance. *Psychology of Sport and Exercise*, 13(5), 533–540.

Gurton, W. H., Matta, G. G., Gough, L. A., & Hurst, P. (2022). Efficacy of sodium bicarbonate ingestion strategies for protecting blinding. *European Journal of Applied Physiology*, 122(12), 2555–2563.

Hopkins, W. G., Hawley, J. A., & Burke, L. M. (1999). Design and analysis of research on sport performance enhancement. *Medicine and Science in Sports and Exercise*, 31(3), 472–485.

Hulston, C. J., & Jeukendrup, A. E. (2009). No placebo effect from carbohydrate intake during prolonged exercise. *International Journal of Sport Nutrition and Exercise Metabolism*, 19(3), 275–284.

Hunter, I., McLeod, A., Valentine, D., Low, T., Ward, J., & Hager, R. (2019). Running economy, mechanics, and marathon racing shoes. *Journal of Sports Sciences*, 37(20), 2367–2373.

Hurst, P., Foad, A., Coleman, D., & Beedie, C. (2017). Athletes intending to use sports supplements are more likely to respond to a placebo. *Medicine & Science in Sports & Exercise (MSSE)*, 49(9), 1877–1883.

Hurst, P., Schipof-Godart, L., Hettinga, F., Roelands, B., & Beedie, C. (2019). Improved 1000-m running performance and pacing strategy with caffeine and placebo: A balanced placebo design study. *International Journal of Sports Physiology and Performance*, 15(4), 483–488.

Hurst, P., Schipof-Godart, L., Szabo, A., Raglin, J., Hettinga, F., Roelands, B., Lane, A., Foad, A., Coleman, D., & Beedie, C. (2020). The placebo and nocebo effect on sports performance: A systematic review. *European Journal of Sport Science*, 20(3), 279–292.

Jones, H. S., Williams, E. L., Bridge, C. A., Marchant, D., Midgley, A. W., Micklewright, D., & Mc Naughton, L. R. (2013). Physiological and psychological effects of deception on pacing strategy and performance: A review. *Sports Medicine*, 43, 1243–1257.

Kalasountas, V., Reed, J., & Fitzpatrick, J. (2007). The effect of placebo-induced changes in expectancies on maximal force production in college students. *Journal of Applied Sport Psychology*, 19(1), 116–124.

Konings, M. J., & Hettinga, F. J. (2018). The impact of different competitive environments on pacing and performance. *International Journal of Sports Physiology and Performance*, 13(6), 701–708.

Lindheimer, J. B., Szabo, A., Raglin, J. S., & Beedie, C. (2020). Advancing the understanding of placebo effects in psychological outcomes of exercise: Lessons learned and future directions. *European Journal of Sport Science*, 20(3), 326–337.

Maganaris, C. N., Collins, D., & Sharp, M. (2000). Expectancy effects and strength training: Do steroids make a difference? *The Sport Psychologist*, 14(3), 272–278.

Marocolo, M., Da Mota, G., Pelegrini, V., & Coriolano, H.-J. A. (2015). Are the beneficial effects of ischemic preconditioning on performance partly a placebo effect? *International Journal of Sports Medicine*, 94(10), 822–825.

McClung, M., & Collins, D. (2007). "Because I know it will!": Placebo effects of an ergogenic aid on athletic performance. *Journal of Sport and Exercise Psychology*, 29(3), 382–394.

Pires, F. O., Dos Anjos, C. A., Covolan, R. J., Fontes, E. B., Noakes, T. D., St Clair Gibson, A., Magalhães, F. H., & Ugrinowitsch, C. (2018). Caffeine and placebo improved maximal exercise performance despite unchanged motor cortex activation and greater prefrontal cortex deoxygenation. *Frontiers in Physiology*, 9, 1144.

Pollo, A., Carlino, E., & Benedetti, F. (2008). The top-down influence of ergogenic placebos on muscle work and fatigue. *European Journal of Neuroscience*, 28(2), 379–388.

Ross, R., Gray, C. M., & Gill, J. M. (2015). The effects of an injected placebo on endurance running performance. *Medicine and Science in Sports and Exercise*, 47(8), 1672–1681.

Rossettini, G., Emadi Andani, M., Dalla Negra, F., Testa, M., Tinazzi, M., & Fiorio, M. (2018). The placebo effect in the motor domain is differently modulated by the external and internal focus of attention. *Scientific Reports*, 8(1), 1–14.

Saunders, B., de Oliveira, L. F., da Silva, R. P., de Salles Painelli, V., Gonçalves, L., Yamaguchi, G., Mutti, T., Maciel, E., Roschel, H., & Artioli, G. (2017). Placebo in sports nutrition: A proof-of-principle study involving caffeine supplementation. *Scandinavian Journal of Medicine & Science in Sports*, 27(11), 1240–1247.

Spencer, M., Bishop, D., Dawson, B., & Goodman, C. (2005). Physiological and metabolic responses of repeated-sprint activities: Specific to field-based team sports. *Sports Medicine, 35*, 1025–1044.

Stone, M., Thomas, K., Wilkinson, M., Jones, A., St Clair Gibson, A., & Thompson, K. (2012). Effects of deception on exercise performance: Implications for determinants of fatigue in humans. *Medicine & Science in Sports & Exercise, 44*(3), 534–541.

Tolusso, D. V., Laurent, C. M., Fullenkamp, A. M., & Tobar, D. A. (2015). Placebo effect: Influence on repeated intermittent sprint performance on consecutive days. *The Journal of Strength & Conditioning Research, 29*(7), 1915–1924.

Williams, E. L., Jones, H. S., Sparks, S. A., Marchant, D. C., Midgley, A. W., & Mc Naughton, L. R. (2015). Competitor presence reduces internal attentional focus and improves 16.1 km cycling time trial performance. *Journal of Science and Medicine in Sport, 18*(4), 486–491.

4

WHAT HAPPENS IN MY BRAIN WHEN I EXPERIENCE A PLACEBO EFFECT?

Neurobiological mechanisms of placebo effects

Bart Roelands

Introduction

Placebo effects don't just happen; rather, they are the result not only of external processes such as information (expectancy) or prior learning (conditioning), but also of the neurobiological response to those external cues. Scientific evidence regarding the mechanism(s) of placebo and nocebo effects is accumulating. This is, however, a complicated quest, as it has also become clear that there is not 'one' placebo effect, but there are many (Ashar et al., 2017). As early as the 1970s there was the acknowledgement that the placebo effect thrives because of neurobiological mechanisms (Beedie et al., 2020; Levine et al., 1978). Since there is no single placebo effect or outcome, it makes sense to accept that there are several distinct and overlapping areas of the brain that are involved in a placebo effect. The onset of a placebo effect is therefore to be found in the complex interplay of different neurobiological pathways and systems. Since scientific knowledge and research techniques are continuously evolving, more and more possibilities to identify potential underlying mechanisms become available.

The role of the brain in the placebo effect can be studied at both the structural and the functional brain levels, with the most commonly used techniques being functional magnetic resonance imaging (fMRI); electro- and magneto-encephalography (EEG and MEG); and positron emission tomography (PET)-based imaging of glucose, dopamine, and opioid activity (Levine et al., 1978). At the same time brain biochemistry should not be ignored, with several important brain neurotransmitters identified as linked to placebo effects. While the placebo effect has mainly been documented in clinical contexts and there is only limited evidence from sports science, an understanding of the full

DOI: 10.4324/9781003229001-4

range of placebo effects and the underpinning mechanisms is important in understanding how placebo effects are likely to influence the effectiveness of interventions in sport (e.g., caffeine, cold-water immersion, altitude training; Roelands & Hurst, 2020).

Brain neurotransmitters involved in the placebo effect

Brain neurotransmitter systems most likely involved in the placebo effect in sport are the opioid, endocannabinoid, and dopamine systems (Beedie et al., 2020). The endogenous opioids (endorphins) are implicated in pain mechanisms (Amanzio & Benedetti, 1999) and respiratory depression (Benedetti et al., 1999). The endocannabinoid system appears to play a pivotal role in placebo analgesia when the opioid system is not involved (Benedetti, Amanzio, et al., 2011). Dopamine is considered pivotal in many movement-related processes such as motivation and reward (Scott et al., 2008).

The opioid system

This system plays an important role in pain mechanisms and respiratory depression. Therefore, the endogenous opioids are an ideal candidate to study the placebo effect. This has mainly been done in clinical settings, but much of this can be related to the sport domain. In one of the first neuroscientific studies of the placebo effect, Levine et al. (1978) showed that pain reduction resulting from the administration of a placebo analgesic could be blocked by naloxone, an opioid antagonist. This suggested that the placebo effect was operating via the same neurobiological pathway as the real analgesic drug it purported to be. Since then, many studies have looked at underlying neural mechanisms of placebo analgesia. Endogenous opioid release has been observed during a sustained pain challenge in several brain structures, including the anterior cingulate cortex (ACC), prefrontal cortex (PFC), insula, amygdala, thalamus and nucleus accumbens (Zubieta et al., 2005). The same group of researchers administered a placebo with the expectation of analgesia during the same pain challenge, and observed endogenous opioid release in several of these regions; the ACC, dorsolateral prefrontal cortex (DLPFC), insula and nucleus accumbens (Zubieta et al., 2005). These studies, and many others, reinforce the earlier suggestion that the placebo treatment often activates the same pathway as the drug that it purports to be (Beedie et al., 2020).

In 2007, Benedetti, Pollo, et al. (2007) took the findings from clinical settings to a different field of research, human performance. Morphine, a powerful analgesic opioid, was used in a simulated sport competition. Subjects had a tourniquet wrapped around their forearm and were required to squeeze a hand-spring exerciser repeatedly until they could no longer continue. Different teams were created and during pre-competition training:

- Teams 1 and 2 trained without any 'drug' administrations
- Teams 3 and 4 were trained with real morphine (note, *not* placebo morphine).
- During an end-of-week competition, Team 1 performed the exercise without treatment, while Teams 2 and Team 3 were administered placebo morphine one hour before competition.
- Team 4 also received a treatment, what they believed was morphine, but which was naloxone, an opioid antagonist (which would be expected to block the opioid pathways).

Data indicated:

- Teams 1 and 2 experienced no placebo effects on performance.
- Team 3 experienced a large placebo effect on pain tolerance following the preconditioning with morphine during the pre-competition phase which they believed been repeated ahead of the competition.
- Team 4 experienced no placebo effects, despite having received morphine in preconditioning trials, they had also received naloxone prior to competition inhibiting the morphine preconditioning effects.

The findings of Benedetti, Pollo, et al. (2007) suggest conditioned activation of endogenous opioids after placebo administration (Benedetti, Lanotte, et al., 2007). Interestingly, these placebo analgesic responses were obtained after only two morphine administrations separated by as much as a week. These findings will be discussed further later in this chapter.

The endocannabinoid system

Pain has often been used as the target variable in placebo effect research. Many studies have focused on the role of the opioid system in the onset and existence of pain. However, repeated (conditioned) exposure to nonsteroidal anti-inflammatory drugs (NSAIDs) as opposed to morphine, appears to generate placebo responses that are not subsequently blocked by naloxone, suggesting that the placebo effect of NSAIDs acts potentially through a different pathway. Research indicates that in NSAID preconditioning it is the endocannabinoid system that is active (Benedetti, Carlino, and Pollo, 2011). Cannabinoids act on cannabinoid receptors located throughout the body but which are most abundant in the brain. There are two types of cannabinoid receptors (1 & 2; CB 1 and CB2), of which CB1 are mostly present in the central nervous system, especially in areas promoting nociception, short-term memory and in the basal ganglia.

Benedetti and his co-workers (Benedetti, Amanzio, et al., 2011) had healthy subjects undergo a pain challenge with the same tourniquet technique they had used in their previous study of performance (Benedetti, Carlino, and Pollo, 2011). The volunteers were divided in six different groups:

- Group 1 underwent a pain tolerance test for four consecutive days (no-treatment control group)
- Group 2 underwent the same procedure as Group 1 but rimonabant, a cannabinoid antagonist, was unbeknownst administered on days 2 and 4
- Group 3 was tested over a period of 5 non-consecutive days. On days 1 and 5, there was no treatment, on days 2 and 3 the subjects were administered morphine as a conditioning drug, and on day 4 the morphine was replaced by placebo without the subjects being aware
- Group 4 underwent the same conditioning as Group 3 but rimonabant was added to the placebo on day 4
- Group 5 followed the same procedure as Group 3 and Group 4 but morphine was replaced by the nonopioid NSAID drug ketorolac (day 4 was placebo)
- Group 6 underwent the same procedure as Group 5 but on day 4 rimonabant was added to the placebo.

The authors reported the following:

- Group 1 experienced no change in pain
- Group 2 experienced no change in pain despite the administration of rimonabant (cannabinoid antagonist).
- Group 3 experienced a direct analgesic effect and reduced pain levels on the days morphine was administered (days 2 and 3), while on day 4 the placebo mimicked the pain responses.
- Group 4 did not experience any change in pain associated with the administration of morphine despite the administration of cannabinoid antagonist rimonabant
- Group 5 experienced significantly higher pain tolerance as the result of the administration of ketorolac
- Group 6 experienced reduced pain tolerance resulting from the inhibition of ketorolac conditioning by the administration rimonabant

Benedetti, Amanzio, et al. (2011) concluded that the findings of this study demonstrate that placebo analgesic responses can be induced by nonopioid pharmacological conditioning with NSAIDs, and that these responses are mediated through the CB1 receptors. Once again, the placebo pathways follow those of the drugs used to condition the response.

From the sports perspective, the studies by Benedetti and colleagues examining the endogenous opioid and endocannabinoid systems are interesting and troubling in equal measure; interesting in that they demonstrate how you can quite predictably generate a quite profound placebo effect on pain and muscular performance, but troubling because – as the authors themselves noted – while illegal drugs were being used to generate the conditioning effect, they were not being used in 'competition', thereby reducing the chances of their use being detected (for further details of links between placebo effects and doping please see chapter 13).

But these studies also use a paradigm that, while no doubt a factor in sports performance as it is in all areas of life, has rarely been used to examine the placebo effect in sport, and that paradigm is conditioning, the systematic development of an association between a stimulus and a response, which harks back to the work of Pavlov over 100 years ago. Perhaps of more relevance to sports performance, and a paradigm more widely used in placebo effect research in sport, is expectancy, the idea that expecting something to happen makes it more likely to happen. For example, if we administer a pill to an athlete and tell them that it's 450mg of caffeine, they will probably have an *expectation* of an effect on their performance (the expectation is not always positive by the way, see the section below and chapter 2). That expectation itself can modify biological processes, and these, in turn, can affect outcomes. Amanzio and Benedetti (1999) argued that expectation triggers endogenous opioids, whereas conditioning activates specific subsystems as we have seen above.

The dopamine system

Another neurotransmitter system associated with the idea of expectation is the dopamine system, with its long-recognised role as the mediator of expectation and reward (Berridge & Kringelbach, 2015). The role of dopamine in the placebo effect has been studied, among other phenomena, in Parkinson's disease patients. De la Fuente-Fernandez (De la Fuente-Fernández et al., 2001) studied the administration of a placebo with the expectation to the patient that the placebo was apomorphine (a dopamine receptor agonist). They observed a significant increase of dopamine release in two areas of the striatum, the ventral (involved in motivation and reward anticipation) and the dorsal (involved in voluntary movement; Lidstone & Stoessl, 2007). Strafella et al. required patients to undergo two PET scans, one at baseline in which there was no treatment, and one experimental scan in which they were told that they has a 50/50% chance of receiving a real treatment, either real or sham repeated Transcranial Magnetic Stimulation (rTMS; Strafella et al., 2006). However, only sham rTMS was administered. Interestingly, the authors found an increased dopamine concentration in the putamen, a brain structure involved in learning and motor control, and also the dopamine concentration in the striatum rose, but failed to reach significance. Lidstone and Stoessl further emphasised the importance of the ventral and the dorsal striatum in the placebo effect. They refer to the study of De la Fuente-Fernández et al. (2001), indicating that all patients had a biochemical response to the placebo treatment, but only half of the patients also showed placebo-induced motor improvements. Interestingly, this group of patients also showed the largest increases in dopamine concentration in the dorsal striatum. The authors further concluded that the increase in dopamine concentration in the ventral striatum, which was observed in all the patients, was related to the patients' expectation of improvement in their symptoms (Lidstone & Stoessl, 2007). Other patient groups have been studied to link the placebo effect to changes in the serotonergic and dopaminergic brain neurotransmitter systems, Volkow et al. (2003) indicated placebo effects when cocaine misusers were administered placebo methylphenidate and Mayberg et al. (2002) studied placebo responses in depressed patients who were administered placebo fluoxetine (selective serotonergic reuptake inhibitor).

The fact that dopamine is involved in the placebo effect from a sport science perspective should not be too much of a surprise. With serotonin, dopamine is heavily implicated in the underlying mechanisms that lead to fatigue – visualised as decrements in performance – during prolonged physical exercise (Meeusen et al., 2021; Roelands & Meeusen, 2010). Fatigue is probably one of the most studied phenomena in sport and exercise science (see also Chapter 5 and 7). It is labelled and debated as a physiologic destination, a perception or emotion, and an important mechanism to minimise physical injury, it is an experimental concept, a symptom, a risk, a cause, and a consequence (Pattyn et al., 2018). Ever since the 1980s the important role of the brain and brain neurotransmission in fatigue has been evident. The original central fatigue hypothesis (Newsholme & Blomstrand, 2006) suggested that an increase in brain serotonin concentration would induce feelings of lethargy and fatigue. This hypothesis was later revised by Davis & Bailey who observed a drop in *dopamine* concentration upon fatigue (Davis & Bailey, 1997). The suggested overlap between the placebo effect and physical fatigue makes fatigue an excellent vehicle to further study the placebo effect in a sport and exercise context.

One additional tool that might lend itself to study neurobiological mechanisms of the placebo effect in sport science is mental fatigue. Mental fatigue can be defined as a psychobiological state caused by prolonged exertion that has the potential to reduce cognitive as well as physical performance (Van Cutsem et al., 2017). After mentally fatiguing tasks, modifications occur in brain EEG activity patterns (i.e. increased activity in the theta, alpha and/or beta). It is postulated that these alterations in brain activity and the concurrent changes in brain neurotransmitter concentrations mediate athletes' perceptions (for example, of mental fatigue) and their drive to exercise (Meeusen et al., 2021; Schiphof-Godart et al., 2018). Although at this moment these are mainly hypothesis and speculations that remain to be confirmed with solid evidence from well-designed scientific studies, there is certainly indirect evidence for a link between mental fatigue and brain neurotransmission. The most frequently suggested, and indirectly studied, neurotransmitters at this stage are dopamine and adenosine, or an interaction of both.

Dopamine, caffeine, and adenosine in placebo caffeine

In a sport science context caffeine has regularly been used as a model to study the placebo effect. The well-known ergogenic effects of caffeine on exercise performance are mainly mediated through central blockade of the adenosine receptors, thereby counteracting the inhibitory effects of adenosine on neuro-excitability, neurotransmitter (dopamine) release and arousal, while there will be a smaller effect due to the metabolic changes induced by caffeine in the periphery (Roelands et al., 2011). Many studies of the placebo effects of caffeine in sports performance have been published; for example, Beedie et al. reported a dose-response relationship in the response to placebo caffeine (Beedie et al., 2006). A group of subjects produced 1.4% less power when they believed they had ingested a placebo, but produced 1.3% more power when they believed to have received a 'low' dose of caffeine (4.5 mg/kg body weight), and over 3% more power when they believed they had received the highest dose of caffeine (9 mg/kg), while in fact an inert placebo was provided on all three occasions. For the reasons described briefly below, it is not easy to examine the mechanisms of these effects in real time in sport. However, these mechanisms have been studies elsewhere. For example, in the first of two studies Kaasinen et al. (2004a) used PET scans to determine that an acute 200 mg dose of caffeine induced significant increases in the dopamine concentration, mainly in the thalamus. In the second study the same authors (Kaasinen et al., 2004b) progressed on their findings to look if the mere expectation of caffeine could lead to dopaminergic effects. Thus, the subjects were aware of the possibility that they would receive either caffeine (200 mg) or placebo (200 mg). They observed that placebo treatment, with the expectation of caffeine, indeed induced changes in the brain dopamine system, specifically in the thalamic region. This might further suggest that placebo drugs are able to activate the same specific brain networks as the pharmacologically active drugs.

Nocebo effects

Nocebo effects, like placebo effects, are underpinned by numerous discrete neurobiological pathways (Tracey, 2010). Expectation of pain has been found to induce nocebo effects observed in the endogenous opioidergic system (Benedetti et al., 2006) and the dopaminergic system (Scott et al., 2008). These nocebo effects involved opposite responses in neurotransmitter systems to responses observed with placebo effects; that is, deactivation of the opioid and dopamine systems. Nocebo effects are also observed in relation to emotional responses such as anxiety; negative verbal suggestions induce antici-patory anxiety, which is associated with the activation of cholecystokinin (CCK), which, in turn, facilitates pain transmission (Benedetti, Lanotte, et al., 2007). The implications of nocebo effects can be significant and long-lasting, with some studies reporting that just one experience of a nocebo effect can influence the efficacy of future treatments (Colloca & Miller, 2011).

Future research

Although more emphasis on the placebo effect in a sport and sport science setting is evident, research into the neurobiological mechanisms by which the effects operate is lacking. In a review by Beedie et al. (2020), several sugges-tions were put forward as to how further exploration could take place. The neurochemical alterations that have been observed and the brain regions, structures and networks that have been identified in clinical settings are yet to be fully translated to the performance context. Imaging of the brain activity by means of electroencephalography (EEG) or functional near-infrared spectros-copy (fNIRS) will be important, but methodological issues such as sweat and movement artefacts and noise have to be solved first. Also, functional mag-netic resonance imaging (fMRI) could aid in highlighting the brain structures involved, but the very small range of movement this allows poses an issue. This could potentially be bypassed by working with expectations of a certain degree of effort or placebo effect, or by assessing cognitive performance and mental fatigue rather than the physical component of fatigue/performance.

Beedie et al. (2020) also suggested that neurotransmitter systems impli-cated in the placebo effect that are also associated with fatigue could be stud-ied via blockade. Given the effects of placebo caffeine have been observed on dopamine pathways of the thalamus and the striatum, theoretically positive effects on performance resulting from dopamine signalling following placebo caffeine administration could be blocked by use of a dopamine antagonist. The same authors, however, cautioned that targeting a single neurotransmitter sys-tem via neurochemical blockade might impact on a number of other brain structures and regions to which that system projects, which are uninvolved in the placebo effect, but which might still be involved in sports performance.

Summary

The current chapter has provided a short overview of the most important brain neurotransmitter systems involved in the placebo effect. Even though much of the research available has been derived from more clinical settings, researchers are more and more engaged in unravelling the role and mechanisms of the pla-cebo effect in a sport and exercise setting. The main neurotransmitters that were identified at this stage are the opioid, endocannabinoid, and dopamine systems.

Certainly, the latter presents the potential to determine the pathways involved in the placebo effect; dopamine concentrations can be manipulated through both pharmacological and nutritional means such as caffeine, with known ergogenic effects. From the available evidence it becomes clear that a substance such as placebo caffeine has the capacity to be ergogenic through the activation of the same specific brain networks as the pharmacologically active drug.

References

Amanzio, M., & Benedetti, F. (1999). Neuropharmacological dissection of placebo analgesia: Expectation-activated opioid systems versus conditioning-activated specific subsystems. *Journal of Neuroscience, 19*(1), 484–494.

Ashar, Y. K., Chang, L. J., & Wager, T. D. (2017). Brain mechanisms of the placebo effect: An affective appraisal account. *Annual Review of Clinical Psychology, 13,* 73–98.

Beedie, C., Benedetti, F., Barbiani, D., Camerone, E., Lindheimer, J., & Roelands, B. (2020). Incorporating methods and findings from neuroscience to better understand placebo and nocebo effects in sport. *European Journal of Sport Science, 20*(3), 313–325.

Beedie, C. J., Stuart, E. M., Coleman, D. A., & Foad, A. J. (2006). Placebo effects of caffeine on cycling performance. *Medicine and Science in Sports and Exercise, 38*(12), 2159.

Benedetti, F., Amanzio, M., Baldi, S., Casadio, C., & Maggi, G. (1999). Inducing placebo respiratory depressant responses in humans via opioid receptors. *European Journal of Neuroscience, 11*(2), 625–631.

Benedetti, F., Amanzio, M., Rosato, R., & Blanchard, C. (2011). Nonopioid placebo analgesia is mediated by CB1 cannabinoid receptors. *Nature Medicine, 17*(10), 1228–1230.

Benedetti, F., Amanzio, M., Vighetti, S., & Asteggiano, G. (2006). The biochemical and neuroendocrine bases of the hyperalgesic nocebo effect. *Journal of Neuroscience, 26*(46), 12014–12022.

Benedetti, F., Carlino, E., & Pollo, A. (2011). How placebos change the patient's brain. *Neuropsychopharmacology, 36*(1), 339–354.

Benedetti, F., Lanotte, M., Lopiano, L., & Colloca, L. (2007). When words are painful: Unraveling the mechanisms of the nocebo effect. *Neuroscience, 147*(2), 260–271.

Benedetti, F., Pollo, A., & Colloca, L. (2007). Opioid-mediated placebo responses boost pain endurance and physical performance: Is it doping in sport competitions? *Journal of Neuroscience, 27*(44), 11934–11939.

Berridge, K. C., & Kringelbach, M. L. (2015). Pleasure systems in the brain. *Neuron, 86*(3), 646–664.

Colloca, L., & Miller, F. G. (2011). The nocebo effect and its relevance for clinical practice. *Psychosomatic Medicine, 73*(7), 598.

Davis, J. M., & Bailey, S. P. (1997). Possible mechanisms of central nervous system fatigue during exercise. *Medicine and Science in Sports and Exercise, 29*(1), 45–57.

De la Fuente-Fernández, R., Ruth, T. J., Sossi, V., Schulzer, M., Calne, D. B., & Stoessl, A. J. (2001). Expectation and dopamine release: Mechanism of the placebo effect in Parkinson's disease. *Science, 293*(5532), 1164–1166.

Kaasinen, V., Aalto, S., Någren, K., & Rinne, J. O. (2004a). Dopaminergic effects of caffeine in the human striatum and thalamus. *Neuroreport, 15*(2), 281–285.

Kaasinen, V., Aalto, S., Någren, K., & Rinne, J. O. (2004b). Expectation of caffeine induces dopaminergic responses in humans. *European Journal of Neuroscience, 19*(8), 2352–2356.

Levine, J., Gordon, N., & Fields, H. (1978). The mechanism of placebo analgesia. *The Lancet, 312*(8091), 654–657.

Lidstone, S. C. C., & Stoessl, A. J. (2007). Understanding the placebo effect: Contributions from neuroimaging. *Molecular Imaging and Biology, 9,* 176–185.

Mayberg, H. S., Silva, J. A., Brannan, S. K., Tekell, J. L., Mahurin, R. K., McGinnis, S., & Jerabek, P. A. (2002). The functional neuroanatomy of the placebo effect. *American Journal of Psychiatry, 159*(5), 728–737.

Meeusen, R., Van Cutsem, J., & Roelands, B. (2021). Endurance exercise-induced and mental fatigue and the brain. *Experimental Physiology, 106*(12), 2294–2298.

Newsholme, E. A., & Blomstrand, E. (2006). Branched-chain amino acids and central fatigue. *The Journal of Nutrition, 136*(1), 274S–276S.

Pattyn, N., Van Cutsem, J., Dessy, E., & Mairesse, O. (2018). Bridging exercise science, cognitive psychology, and medical practice: Is "cognitive fatigue" a remake of "the emperor's new clothes"? *Frontiers in Psychology, 9,* 1246.

Roelands, B., Buyse, L., Pauwels, F., Delbeke, F., Deventer, K., & Meeusen, R. (2011). No effect of caffeine on exercise performance in high ambient temperature. *European Journal of Applied Physiology, 111,* 3089–3095.

Roelands, B., & Hurst, P. (2020). The placebo effect in sport: How practitioners can inject words to improve performance. *International Journal of Sports Physiology and Performance, 15*(6), 765–766.

Roelands, B., & Meeusen, R. (2010). Alterations in central fatigue by pharmacological manipulations of neurotransmitters in normal and high ambient temperature. *Sports Medicine, 40,* 229–246.

Schiphof-Godart, L., Roelands, B., & Hettinga, F. J. (2018). Drive in sports: How mental fatigue affects endurance performance. *Frontiers in Psychology, 9,* 1383.

Scott, D. J., Stohler, C. S., Egnatuk, C. M., Wang, H., Koeppe, R. A., & Zubieta, J.-K. (2008). Placebo and nocebo effects are defined by opposite opioid and dopaminergic responses. *Archives of General Psychiatry, 65*(2), 220–231.

Strafella, A. P., Ko, J. H., & Monchi, O. (2006). Therapeutic application of transcranial magnetic stimulation in Parkinson's disease: The contribution of expectation. *NeuroImage, 31*(4), 1666–1672.

Tracey, I. (2010). Getting the pain you expect: Mechanisms of placebo, nocebo and reappraisal effects in humans. *Nature Medicine, 16*(11), 1277.

Van Cutsem, J., Marcora, S., De Pauw, K., Bailey, S., Meeusen, R., & Roelands, B. (2017). The effects of mental fatigue on physical performance: A systematic review. *Sports Medicine, 47*(8), 1569–1588.

Volkow, N. D., Fowler, J. S., & Wang, G.-J. (2003). The addicted human brain: Insights from imaging studies. *The Journal of Clinical Investigation, 111*(10), 1444–1451.

Zubieta, J.-K., Bueller, J. A., Jackson, L. R., Scott, D. J., Xu, Y., Koeppe, R. A., Nichols, T. E., & Stohler, C. S. (2005). Placebo effects mediated by endogenous opioid activity on μ-opioid receptors. *Journal of Neuroscience, 25*(34), 7754–7762.

5

ARE PLACEBO EFFECTS SPECIAL?

A social-evolutionary perspective on resource perception in exercise-induced fatigue and performance

Emma Cohen

Introduction

Placebo effects in health and exercise contexts are broadly understood as biobehavioural effects of positive expectations about treatments and ergogenic aids. Clinical studies operationalise placebo as a fake medical treatment, while studies of placebo effects in sport and exercise typically administer a fake performance aid (e.g., nutritional, mechanical; Hurst et al., 2020). In neuroscience and psychology, it is widely understood that it is not the treatment per se that produces effects, nor are effects "all in the mind". Rather, effects are engendered though integrated cognitive, emotional, physiological and behavioural responses (Benedetti, 2021). Specifically, (implicit or explicit) expectancy has become central to causal accounts of placebo effects, and mechanistic pathways from expectancy to effect are increasingly understood through modern physiological and neuroscientific methods and tools (Tracey, 2010).

Recent studies have revealed overlapping neurophysiological mechanisms involved in placebo effects and other exogenously induced effects, offering clues to functional continuities among phenomena traditionally viewed as distinct. For example, expectations of treatment efficacy and perceptions of social support appear to be functionally homologous through their common associations with threat attenuation, safety, and resource availability, and mechanistically continuous through their common activation of opioidergic and endocannabinoid systems and neural reward and threat response circuitry (Shamay-Tsoory & Eisenberger, 2021; Wager et al., 2007). In light of these recent advances, it is reasonable to question the value of "placebo", traditionally defined, as a distinct category in causal analysis. Indeed, the conceptual separation of placebo effects from functionally and mechanistically similar

DOI: 10.4324/9781003229001-5

expectancy-derived effects appears to be more strongly anchored in cultural tradition than recent science, hampering systematic cross-cultural, cross-domain and cross-disciplinary investigation.

This chapter attempts to situate the traditional notion of placebo in its proper causal context – evolutionary, psychological, physiological and ecological. The concept of placebo will be reappraised in light of recent findings from evolutionary anthropology to social neuroscience. Specifically, placebo effects in sport and exercise are reconceptualised within an evolutionary framework of brain–body homeostatic regulation that integrates implicit and explicit perception of interoceptive and exteroceptive states. Whereas homeostasis is traditionally thought to entail the automatic regulation of functional operations, the broader approach adopted here recognises, following Damasio (2019), that sensations and "feelings are the subjective experiences of the state of life – that is, of homeostasis – in all creatures endowed with a mind and a conscious point of view" (p. 25) and that individuals and socio-cultural groups "can both interfere with automatic regulatory mechanisms *and* create new forms of life regulation" (p. 46) via social relationships, symbolic culture and cultural evolution (Humphrey & Skoyles, 2012). In this view, homeostatic regulation is mediated by socially and culturally situated affect, offering a useful framework for thinking about how positively valenced expectancy in placebo settings influences physiological function.

As a case study, we will consider the role of perceived fatigue in endurance performance. Exercise-induced fatigue is here defined as a progressive decline in the ability to continue a given exercise. Our focus will be on the role of the subjective experience of fatigue as part of a whole-body regulatory process (Marino, 2019) of dynamic, adaptive calibration to internal and external conditions, considering, in particular, (perceived) resource availability. Among many other factors, perceptions of available resources (e.g., via ergogenic aids) modulate sensations of fatigue (Pollo et al., 2008). In turn, these hard-to-ignore sensations of tiredness and increasing effort are a crucial limiting – or protective – homeostatic factor in performance. Sensations of fatigue and effort therefore link expectancies about available resources and performance. Like perceptions of pain, they are dynamically calibrated within a complex interoceptive and exteroceptive ecology, including not just the physical environment but also the social environment (Noakes, 2012; Noakes et al., 2005; St Clair Gibson et al., 2017).

Although it is now broadly accepted that perceptions of social support can profoundly influence psychophysiological regulation and health, this observation has yet to penetrate the scientific study of fatigue and performance (Davis & Cohen, 2018; Davis, Crittenden, et al., 2021). The argument advanced here is that, whether implicit or explicit and whether elicited through social cues or perceived treatments, expectancies of exogenous support and resource play a significant role in psychophysiological regulation of energy, fatigue, and performance. Social support is here broadly construed to refer to the extent to which an individual has (or perceived themselves to have) access to bio-energetic resources and care from/via others. This perspective challenges and reframes the superficial placebo/non-placebo distinction and connects expectancies associated with perceived treatments and social context within a unifying evolutionary framework. The focus on resource expectancy as a crucial element in adaptive energy regulation and endurance performance also complements and balances the predominant focus in exercise psychology on motivational factors.

Adaptively calibrated fatigue and performance

The concept of placebo has an enduring and alluring hold on intuitive, or folk, psychology – specifically, the dualistic notion that the stuff of the mind (e.g., perception, belief) is separate from the stuff of the body (e.g., physiology, immune function; Cohen et al., 2011). Placebo effects violate this assumption and, like many other counterintuitive ideas that pervade and persist in culture, this potentially contributes to their intrinsic appeal (Boyer, 2008). Modern cognitive science rejects this dualism, however, and replaces it with a view of mind, body and environment as dynamically linked in homeostatic function. In this context, perceptions and sensations play an integral role in the "homeostatic imperative" that sustains life (Damasio, 2019). It follows that placebo effects, although potentially counterintuitive, are not particularly special. Rather, they are the natural and expected outcome of a system of dynamic homeostatic regulation that admits perceptions, beliefs, expectations, hopes, sensations, and feelings.

Whereas placebo effects were traditionally understood and dismissed as being "all in the mind", early scientific perspectives on fatigue in exercise broadly viewed it as being "all in the body". In this perspective, the highly motivated but exhausted athlete slows down and ultimately stops on reaching a critical threshold of peripheral fatigue, a metabolic end-point (Marino, 2019). Now, however, there is wide acknowledgement of the integrative and regulatory role of the central nervous system in perceived fatigue and endurance performance. In recent multidimensional models, fatigue is neither all in the mind nor all in the body. Perceptions of fatigue regulate behaviour and are themselves constructed in any given moment within a complex interoceptive and exteroceptive ecology (Marcora, 2019; St Clair Gibson et al., 2017). Notably, although recent approaches have elevated the role of the brain in exercise performance, this has not entailed a wholesale pendulum swing to a neurocentric or neuroessentialist view, with the brain exaggerated as controller of the body and the complete material basis of the mind. The immediate importance of embodied homeostatic regulation in pacing and performance in exercise supports a view of the brain as an "organ of interrelations" between the living organism and its natural environment (Fuchs, 2017) and as "a servant of whole-organism homeostasis"(Damasio, 2019, p. 64).

From an evolutionary perspective, sensations of fatigue are thought to be part of an energy regulation strategy that maintains expenditure within safe limits (Marino, 2019). Natural selection has tended to favour organisms that can efficiently manage their limited energetic resources across fitness-relevant activities (physical activity, reproduction, immune function, etc.) (Pontzer & McGrosky, 2022). Although it is intuitive to consider endurance exercise in terms of energy *expenditure*, the focus on adaptive regulation equally reminds us of the importance of strategic energy *conservation*. In this context, sensations of fatigue (like pain) are commonly understood to serve a protective function; they contribute to the adaptive maintenance of a functional "reserve", crucial for optimising survival chances in "extraordinary moments" (Marino, 2019, p. 95). It follows that the adaptively determined reserve is not a static value but is flexibly calibrated to relevant parameters of the exercise context, from the perceived strategic value of the exercise goal (e.g., Olympic gold medal) to the competing energetic requirements across different fitness-relevant domains (e.g., immune, reproductive) an athlete presents on a given occasion. Depending on this very broad range of conditions, sensations of fatigue – the homeostatic alarm system – will be felt more or less intensely for a given physiological effort (Noakes, 2012).

This adaptive calibration/conservation account posits that the association between perceived fatigue and a given energetic expenditure or performance output are not fixed (irrespective of any potential efficiency factors at play). Analogous to the relationship between nociceptive input and perceived pain, the relationship between energetic expenditure and perceived fatigue is not one-to-one, but is tuned to a range of conditions (Tracey, 2010). At the cognitive level, these include and integrate feelings and beliefs about the strategic benefit or reward of the exercise (i.e., motivational factors), feelings and beliefs about any factor that is potentially associated with risk, threat or cost of the activity (e.g., injury, task duration), and feelings and beliefs about available energetic resources that can be budgeted to the activity (Marcora, 2019; St Clair Gibson et al., 2017).

Whereas a vast amount of research across a diverse range of paradigms – from self-talk to false-feedback – has focused on performance effects of motivation and perceived threat or cost, relatively less is known about the effects of perceived resource availability on energy regulation, fatigue, and performance. However, two separate bodies of work – on carbohydrate mouth-rinsing and ergogenic placebos – offer support for the integral role of resource expectancy in fatigue and performance. For example, studies on carbohydrate mouth-rinsing have reported significantly improved performance in cycling time-trials (vs. rinsing with water) in the absence of any significant increase in perceived exertion (Carter et al., 2004). Similarly, performance effects of perceived nutritional aids have been demonstrated across a large body of research on placebo effects (Beedie et al., 2006; Pollo et al., 2008). For example, Beedie et al. (2006) reported a 3.1% (SD = 3.4%) mean improvement relative to baseline when participants were told they had received a high dose of caffeine, without corresponding increases in physiological load, and a 1.4% (SD = 3.1%) performance decline when they were told they had received a placebo. Feedback from participants included "I was able to push harder with less pain", "It was easier to put the effort in, there wasn't any tiredness creeping in", and "I thought 'this is a damn sight easier than it was the last time'". The results and qualitative statements are consistent with the hypothesis that perceptions of available ergogenic resources can relax the energetic safety margin, reduce sensations of fatigue or perceived exertion and increase performance output via expectancy-derived adaptive calibration (see also Benedetti et al., 2018).

In summary, sensations of fatigue are a response to a range of conditions within and beyond the body. They reflect (in part) a dynamic adaptive response to current and anticipated conditions of energetic demand and supply and, via their effects on behaviour, are a crucial factor in energy regulation. Perceived fatigue and performance in exercise do not only reflect how much energy is (thought to be) available, but how much energy is strategically conserved to successfully and safely meet current and future demands across the full range of energetic domains (e.g., maintenance and recovery, immunity, reproduction, physical activity). Better performance is therefore not only about "pushing harder" (i.e., motivation) but creating the conditions that calibrate these systems to *conserve less* (Marino, 2019). Motivations around the value of the exercise goal are just part of this equation. Perceptions of task duration (i.e., energetic requirements) and available resources also play a crucial role in energy regulation, sensations of fatigue and performance.

Clearly, this calibration largely takes place outside conscious awareness, and factors affecting it are not all necessarily perceived or understood explicitly. Studies on placebo ergogenic aids suggest that explicit expectations about available resources influence adaptive energy regulation, improving performance for a given level of perceived fatigue and effort. However, these studies represent a narrow slice of potentially relevant conditions; environmental cues to energetic resources may also be perceived implicitly as well as indirectly (through associational learning). Although not normally studied for their effects on performance physiology, cooperative social relationships represent one of the most salient factors associated with energetic availability in humans. As such, perceived social support shares a fundamental continuity with perceived ergogenic support in that both signal access to resources relevant for task completion and recovery.

Perceived social support as a cue to energetic resource

Sociality... is part of the toolkit of homeostasis

(Damasio, 2019, p. 114)

Across evolutionary and developmental timespans, the energetic resources that sustain human life and health are channelled through social relationships characterised by long-term social bonds (Hrdy, 2009). Adaptations to this social ecology include abilities to track potential opportunities as well as threats, and to solicit support, care and other resources (Tomasello et al., 2012). Socially bonded and supportive others can therefore represent a cue to energy availability, with potential for homeostatic effects on energy regulation and performance that are comparable to perceived nutritional aids. Neuro-scientific research suggests that cues to close attachment figures are correlated with attenuation of pain responses and associated activity in pain-processing networks and with increased neural activity in areas associated with safety signalling (Eisenberger et al., 2011). An adaptive approach to performance regulation should similarly clarify the modulating effect of social support – a potentially salient cue of safety and resource, and a pervasive element in sport settings (e.g., through team-mates, coaches, fans) – on perceived fatigue, energy regulation and performance.

Although recent exercise science has made significant progress toward an integrative brain–body understanding of the limits of human performance (see also Chapter 7), the discussion remains resolutely individualistic. Consideration of relevant social factors and how they relate to the perception of available resources, and therefore performance, is largely limited to social-motivational factors having to do with competition, not cooperation or perceptions of support. Early studies on "social facilitation", originating in the early observations of Norman Triplett in the late 19th century, demonstrated that social presence enhanced simple task performance but impaired complex task performance (Aiello & Douthitt, 2001). Subsequently, following Cottrell's social evaluation account of facilitation effects (beyond "mere presence") (Cottrell, 1972), the bulk of research focused on anxiety-related reactions to potentially evaluative and threatening social presence. In this paradigm, mechanistic explanations have emphasised arousal, evaluation apprehension, and distraction caused by the presence of others.

In contrast, evolutionary anthropology situates and examines uniquely human capacities for endurance performance in the context of the "Metabolic Revolution" that accompanied the emergence of hominin cooperative foraging, and which Herman Pontzer has pithily summarised as involving co-evolution among "sharing, smarts, and stamina" (Pontzer, 2021, p. 137).

Just as survival and reproduction became increasingly dependent on energetically richer foods through novel forms of cooperative foraging, so too were they increasingly tied to close, supportive relationships with others. Close relationships would come to signify resource availability, and the resource pooling and sharing that occurred via such relationships would have profoundly influenced adaptive strategies of energy expenditure and allocation in everyday activity, from persistence hunting to immunity. The human capacity for endurance activity – unique among primates – is therefore evolutionarily yoked to our capacity for sharing energetic resources, directly in the form of food but also buffering risk through provision of care.

In clinical studies, the fitness-relevant impact of social connections and support (e.g., on stress, immune function, longevity) is increasingly recognised, with *perceived* support predicting outcomes more reliably than *received* support (Cohen & Wills, 1985; Zimet et al., 1988). Integrating the evolutionary literatures on fatigue and cooperation, it can be hypothesised that a similarly important role arises for perceived social resources in strategic energetic expenditure/conservation in exercise, and in subjective experiences of effort and fatigue. Just as expectancies about ergogenic aids appear to allow access to biological reserves, expectancies of additional resource availability via social cues can potentially relax the safety margin that regulates energy expenditure, allowing more endogenous resources to be delivered and utilised in the exercise activity (all else being equal, such as motivational factors). Accordingly, cues to social safety, whether implicitly or explicitly perceived, modulate and calibrate sensations – or "alarms" – of fatigue. In the context of these cues, for a given increase in energy expenditure, sensations of fatigue are not similarly heightened. That is, for a given level of perceived fatigue, energetic expenditure and performance are increased relative to conditions of social isolation or perceived lack of social support.

Recent studies offer some preliminary support for this account. For example, we have observed social ergogenic effects on performance and perceptions of pain, fatigue and energy across a range of exercise contexts (Cohen et al., 2010; Davis & Cohen, 2018; Davis et al., 2015; Davis, Crittenden, et al., 2021; Davis, MacCarron, et al., 2021; Tarr et al., 2015). Social ergogenic effects were variously engendered through cues of social bonding (e.g., behaviourally synchronous warm-up), cues of attachment figure (e.g., photograph), and perceived social connection and integration. In running trials (Davis et al., 2015) and hand-grip tasks (Davis, Crittenden, et al., 2021), increased performance was observed for the same or lower perceived exertion in conditions that cued social bonds and support, and social ergogenic effects were stronger under objectively more difficult conditions (i.e., where resource needs were greatest). Social factors relating to positive relationships and community support and integration also indirectly predicted better performance (faster 5-km run times) via increased perceived energy in a sample of Parkrun participants

(Davis, MacCarron, et al., 2021). While social facilitation and other motivational factors may also be at play, findings are consistent with the hypothesis that cooperative sociality relaxes the safety margin that conserves energy for deployment in other activities. By this account, the isolated and unsupported athlete is potentially not just less motivated; they are less able to access their protective reserve of energy.

Functional homology of ergogenic placebos and perceived support (or, why placebo effects aren't special)

The adaptive calibration account of energy, fatigue and performance regulation unifies placebos and social support via their shared role in resource expectancy. Beliefs and expectancies about available resources, in turn, influence homeostatic regulation of energy expenditure. Cues associated with resource availability will, all else being equal, allow a less precautionary approach to the conservation of biological reserve, reflected in reduced sensations of fatigue and greater performance outputs. In this account, cues to social support and cues to ergogenic aids are not just analogous, but functionally homologous, an understanding hitherto inhibited by the arbitrary divides of mind–body dualism and academic tradition. Dissociating these as placebo and not-placebo prioritises the trigger over the cause, arbitrarily separates entire fields of enquiry (e.g., clinical neuroscience and social neuroscience) and glosses deeper functional commonalities in how these factors function (e.g., via perceptions of safety and resource availability). Reconceptualising placebo in terms of evolved homeostatic function and, more specifically, in terms of perceptions of safety and resource availability identifies a more fundamental continuity between perceived social support, ergogenic aids and fake treatments – all signal presence of resource and, relative to their absence, a reduction of risk. All else being equal, this permits a less precautionary strategy in the utilisation/conservation of energetic stores.

Further research is needed to test this account and to establish the hypothesised causal links from perceived social resource to sensations of fatigue and performance outputs via adaptive energy regulation. Comparisons across forms of resource expectancy would determine the value of the framework generally for unifying disparate strands of research within an adaptive regulation framework. Pain research (Bingel et al., 2011; Eisenberger et al., 2011) has shown that analgesia can be induced both through expectations of treatment efficacy (placebo effects) and through perceptions of social support via overlapping neurophysiological pathways (e.g., endocannabinoid, opioidergic; safety signalling). Similar research on energy expenditure and perceived fatigue in endurance activity across placebo and social support contexts could help determine mechanistic continuities and test hypothesised links to safety signalling (Davis, Crittenden, et al., 2021). Systematic approaches could further investigate synergies and trade-offs among crucial cognitive factors in the homeostatic regulation of fatigue, chiefly perceived resources, perceived demands, and motivations. Mechanical and ergogenic placebos could be integrated within a systematic comparison of placebo interventions targeting perceived demand and perceived resource, respectively. The implications of this account for the co-evolution of human sociality and energetics have also yet to be developed and explored. For example, cooperative sociality may have buffered the energetic risks of endurance running for persistence hunting, allowing energy conservation in endurance activity to be less cautious, and potentially facilitating the evolution of this behavioural strategy. Further, individual differences in responses to socially cues should be explored. Just as studies of placebo effects have distinguished between responders and non-responders, studies of social support effects report variation in response to social cues. The account presented here predicts that individual variation in the ergogenic response to social cues in part reflects variation in experiences of social support. For example, if a child has limited opportunities to associate social support figures or social relationships with resource availability and sharing throughout development, the link to safety and resource perception would be relatively weaker than among individuals for whom such opportunities are frequent.

Conclusion

Definitions of placebo are typically narrowly construed in terms of explicit or conditioned beliefs about the efficacy of a given "fake" treatment. However, whether beliefs, perceptions, sensations and expectancies are based on fakery or not is of little relevance to their function in homeostatic processes that regulate energy, behaviour and life. The study of dynamically adaptive, protective, psychobiological functions, such as fatigue, in evolutionary, social, and developmental context helps reconceptualise placebo effects as a normal part of neurally-mediated homeostasis that admits perceptions, sensations and expectancies about perceived task demands as well as perceived resources and support, and that serves to maintain activity levels within safe limits (Damasio, 2019; Marino, 2019). In humans, energetic requirements are delivered via intense caregiver relationships throughout our long period of developmental dependency and via cooperative relationships throughout the lifespan (Hrdy, 2009). Dynamic energy regulation is therefore conditioned and calibrated not just to biological and physical conditions, but also importantly within a cooperative social ecology. While energy cannot literally be drawn from fans in stands or fake pills, the adaptive calibration account posits that cues of (socially mediated) resource availability can inhibit energy conservation, moderate fatigue, and boost performance. The power of the "12th man", like the power of placebo, may therefore be greater than we have realised.

Acknowledgements

Thanks to Arran Davis for comments on a previous version of this chapter, and to members of the Social Body Lab for helpful discussions. This research is supported by a James S. McDonnell Foundation 21st Century Science Initiative Understanding Human Cognition Opportunity Award (10.37717/2020-1152).

References

Aiello, J. R., & Douthitt, E. A. (2001). Social facilitation from triplett to electronic performance monitoring. *Group Dynamics: Theory, Research, and Practice, 5*(3), 163–180. https://doi.org/10.1037/1089-2699.5.3.163

Beedie, C. J., Stuart, E. M., Coleman, D. A., & Foad, A. J. (2006). Placebo effects of caffeine on cycling performance. *Medicine and Science in Sports and Exercise, 38*(12), 2159.

Benedetti, F. (2021). Placebos and movies: What do they have in common? *Current Directions in Psychological Science, 30*(3), 274–279. https://doi.org/10.1177/09637214211003892

Benedetti, F., Barbiani, D., & Camerone, E. (2018). Critical life functions: Can placebo replace oxygen? *International Review of Neurobiology, 138*, 201–218.

Bingel, U., Wanigasekera, V., Wiech, K., Ni Mhuircheartaigh, R., Lee, M. C., Ploner, M., & Tracey, I. (2011). The effect of treatment expectation on drug efficacy: Imaging the analgesic benefit of the opioid remifentanil. *Science Translational Medicine, 3*(70), 70ra14.

Boyer, P. (2008). *Religion explained*. Random House.

Carter, J. M., Jeukendrup, A. E., & Jones, D. A. (2004). The effect of carbohydrate mouth rinse on 1-h cycle time trial performance. *Medicine & Science in Sports & Exercise, 36*(12), 2107–2111. https://doi.org/10.1249/01.mss.0000147585.65709.6f PMID - 15570147

Cohen, E., Burdett, E., Knight, N., & Barrett, J. (2011). Cross-cultural similarities and differences in person-body reasoning: Experimental Evidence From the United Kingdom and Brazilian Amazon. *Cognitive Science, 35*(7), 1282–1304. https://doi.org/10.1111/j.1551-6709.2011.01172.x PMID - 21884221

Cohen, E., Ejsmond-Frey, R., Knight, N., & Dunbar, R. I. (2010). Rowers' high: Behavioural synchrony is correlated with elevated pain thresholds. *Biology Letters, 6*(1), 106–108.

Cohen, S., & Wills, T. A. (1985). Stress, social support, and the buffering hypothesis. *Psychological Bulletin, 98*(2), 310–357. https://doi.org/10.1037/0033-2909.98.2.310

Cottrell, N. B. (1972). Social facilitation. *Experimental Social Psychology, 185*, 236.

Damasio, A. (2019). *The strange order of things: Life feeling and the making of cultures*. Pantheon Books.

Davis, A., & Cohen, E. (2018). The effects of social support on strenuous physical exercise. *Adaptive Human Behavior and Physiology, 4*(2), 171–187.

Davis, A., Taylor, J., & Cohen, E. (2015). Social bonds and exercise: Evidence for a reciprocal relationship. *PLoS One, 10*(8), e0136705. https://doi.org/10.1371/journal.pone.0136705.s012

Davis, A. J., Crittenden, B., & Cohen, E. (2021). Effects of social support on performance outputs and perceived difficulty during physical exercise. *Physiology & Behavior*, *239*, 113490.

Davis, A. J., MacCarron, P., & Cohen, E. (2021). Social reward and support effects on exercise experiences and performance: Evidence from Parkrun. *PLoS One*, *16*(9), e0256546.

Eisenberger, N. I., Master, S. L., Inagaki, T. K., Taylor, S. E., Shirinyan, D., Lieberman, M. D., & Naliboff, B. D. (2011). Attachment figures activate a safety signal-related neural region and reduce pain experience. *Proceedings of the National Academy of Sciences*, *108*(28), 11721–11726. https://doi.org/10.1073/pnas.1108239108

Fuchs, T. (2017). *Ecology of the brain: The phenomenology and biology of the embodied mind*. Oxford University Press.

St Clair Gibson, A., Swart, J., & Tucker, R. (2017). The interaction of psychological and physiological homeostatic drives and role of general control principles in the regulation of physiological systems, exercise and the fatigue process – The integrative governor theory. *European Journal of Sport Science*, *18*(1), 25–36. https://doi.org/10.1080/17461391.2017.1321688 PMID - 28478704

Hrdy, S. B. (2009). *Mothers and others: The evolutionary origins of mutual understanding*. Harvard University Press.

Humphrey, N., & Skoyles, J. (2012). The evolutionary psychology of healing: A human success story. *Current Biology*, *22*(17), R695–R698.

Hurst, P., Schipof-Godart, L., Szabo, A., Raglin, J., Hettinga, F., Roelands, B., Lane, A., Foad, A., Coleman, D., & Beedie, C. (2020). The placebo and nocebo effect on sports performance: A systematic review. *European Journal of Sport Science*, *20*(3), 279–292.

Marcora, S. (2019). Psychobiology of fatigue during endurance exercise. In C. Meijen (Ed.), *Endurance performance in sport: Psychological theory and interventions* (pp. 15–34). Routledge.

Marino, F. E. (2019). *Human fatigue: Evolution, health and performance*. Routledge.

Noakes, T. D. (2012). Fatigue is a brain-derived emotion that regulates the exercise behavior to ensure the protection of whole body homeostasis. *Frontiers in Physiology*, *3*(82), 1–13. https://doi.org/10.3389/fphys.2012.00082

Noakes, T. D., St Clair Gibson, A., & Lambert, E. V. (2005). From catastrophe to complexity: A novel model of integrative central neural regulation of effort and fatigue during exercise in humans: Summary and conclusions. *British Journal of Sports Medicine*, *39*(2), 120–124.

Pollo, A., Carlino, E., & Benedetti, F. (2008). The top-down influence of ergogenic placebos on muscle work and fatigue. *European Journal of Neuroscience*, *28*(2), 379–388.

Pontzer, H. (2021). *Burn: The misunderstood science of metabolism*. Penguin UK.

Pontzer, H., & McGrosky, A. (2022). Balancing growth, reproduction, maintenance, and activity in evolved energy economies. *Current Biology*, *32*(12), R709–R719. https://doi.org/10.1016/j.cub.2022.05.018 PMID - 35728556

Shamay-Tsoory, S. G., & Eisenberger, N. I. (2021). Getting in touch: A neural model of comforting touch. *Neuroscience & Biobehavioral Reviews*, *130*, 263–273. https://doi.org/10.1016/j.neubiorev.2021.08.030

Tarr, B., Launay, J., Cohen, E., & Dunbar, R. (2015). Synchrony and exertion during dance independently raise pain threshold and encourage social bonding. *Biology Letters*, *11*(10), 20150767. https://doi.org/10.1098/rsbl.2015.0767

Tomasello, M., Melis, A. P., Tennie, C., Wyman, E., & Herrmann, E. (2012). Two key steps in the evolution of human cooperation: The interdependence hypothesis. *Current Anthropology*, *53*(6), 673–692. https://doi.org/10.1086/668207

Tracey, I. (2010). Getting the pain you expect: Mechanisms of placebo, nocebo and reappraisal effects in humans. *Nature Medicine*, *16*(11), 1277.

Wager, T. D., Scott, D. J., & Zubieta, J.-K. (2007). Placebo effects on human μ-opioid activity during pain. *Proceedings of the National Academy of Sciences*, *104*(26), 11056–11061.

Zimet, G. D., Dahlem, N. W., Zimet, S. G., & Farley, G. K. (1988). The multidimensional scale of perceived social support. *Journal of Personality Assessment*, *52*(1), 30–41.

6

DO I THINK OR DO I FEEL A PLACEBO EFFECT?

Placebo effects and emotion in sport

Chris Beedie

Before we begin, I would like you to consider this scenario:

> Judy is about to compete in the biggest race of her life. She is extremely nervous. During the warm-up her coach says, "I'm going to tell you something I've never told you before." On hearing this Judy feels her anxiety building even more. Her coach continues, "For the last month I've been lying to you about your race time; every session you did I said you were about one second slower than was the case. I did this because I want you to be hungry for this win and to train as hard as you can. But it means that you can trust me when I say that you will run faster today than you thought you would."

After getting over the shock, Judy's nervous anxiety initially turns to confusion and then to hope and then to excitement. And the coach's prediction was accurate; Judy had the best race of her life, produced her fastest-ever time, and won the event. But even so she was a bit angry with her coach, and after she'd cooled down from the race, she asked him why he'd felt it necessary to lie to her for over a month. He replied that he'd only lied once, and that it was 90 minutes ago, during the warm-up. He said he could see how anxious she was and felt he needed to do something to calm her down. He'd read that such 'placebo effects' can significantly enhance sports performance, and knowing Judy well, thought that it was likely to be effective, even though it is something that he could probably only ever do the one time.

DOI: 10.4324/9781003229001-6

The above might seem a little unusual, even unethical (see the chapter by Campos et al. in this book) but situations like these happen frequently in sport, and indeed in life more generally. Here are some questions about the above vignette that you might want to think about before you read this chapter:

1. Is it possible that simply being told that she was going to run faster could make Judy run faster?
2. If the answer to Question 1 is 'Yes', what was the mechanism? What has changed that allows Judy to produce a personal best time?
3. What role might Judy's emotional responses, which travelled from nervousness, to anxiety, to shock, to hope, and to excitement, have played in her apparently optimal performance?

Introduction

I've been studying placebo effects in sport for over 20 years. I can't count how many times athletes, coaches, and even scientists have said to me "The placebo effect is amazing." I also can't count how many times those same people have looked a little disappointed when instead of my agreeing enthusiastically, I've replied "It really isn't, it's just routine and predictable biology." The same is true of emotion. And these are ideas I would like you to keep in mind as you read this chapter.

A placebo effect is a positive outcome resulting from the belief that a beneficial treatment has been received or that greater resources are available to the athlete than they initially believed. Placebo effects based on deceptive information have been found to improve the performance of athletes in a wide range of sports (Beedie & Foad, 2009; Hurst et al., 2020). Whilst most empirical research in sport has focussed on nutritional placebos (Hurst et al., 2020), it is recognised that the simple spoken word can also elicit a placebo effect (Davis et al., 2020). In fact, given that most placebo effects appear to be the result of deliberately or inadvertently modified expectation, arguably any intervention that can modify expectations in a positive direction can, in the right circumstances, also elicit a placebo effect. In this chapter, it will be argued that the degree to which the modified expectation also modifies an athlete's emotions is also a critical factor.

Background

To date the placebo effect has been studied in sport as a standalone phenomenon and has not been incorporated into any broader theories or models. Perhaps as a result, either of two extreme views tend to characterise people's thoughts about the placebo effect in sport:

1. The placebo effect is a fake idea, an illusory construct resulting from poor data analysis or from the failure of the athletes, practitioners, or scientists involved to appreciate and understand the *real* mechanisms underlying what *appear* to be placebo effects. Such mechanisms might range from regression to the mean to voluntary changes in effort and motivation to random or systematic biological variation.
2. It is a quasi-magical phenomenon, evidence that the human psyche or spirit can produce effects that defy logic, science, or even nature, something more akin to the supernatural than to nature as science understands it.

The scientific reality is, of course, far closer to the first, although given the way it can be portrayed in the media the placebo effect can certainly appear to be closer to the second. Placebo effects, while being a real and unique phenomenon in some respects, are in real terms simply part and parcel of a broader category of implicit/evolved and explicit/acquired self-regulatory processes, including but not limited to homeostasis, chronobiology, emotion, mood, and self-control (Lieberman, 2006). This chapter examines placebo effects within this broader category and links these effects specifically to emotion with the aim of helping those involved in all areas of sport, from athlete to scientist, to understand the overlap between placebo effects about which we know relatively little, and emotion about which we know a lot.

The rationale for this attempt is simple. Placebo effects, like emotions, do not happen in isolation, they happen within human nervous & endocrine systems engineered by millions of years of evolution to be economic and efficient. It simply doesn't make sense in evolutionary terms that humans (and other species) would carry a discrete and independent placebo response system (see Chapter 5). In the same way that emotions use the existing circuitry of the nervous and endocrine systems – and to a large degree of the entire body – to generate powerful biasing effects on brain and behaviour, so do placebo effects.

Emotion in sport

Sport is an emotional thing. When we think of sport from all sides of the process; competitors (and their families), coaches and other non-playing support staff, audiences, commentators, journalists, officials, sponsors, and owners, all tend to experience and often express emotions, and these are often quite extreme emotions by comparison with those they express in relation to their non-sporting lives. The ecstasy and joy of victory, the pain of defeat, anxiety before a final, relief when it's over, remorse over a missed opportunity, shame at letting the side down, fear of injury, sadness at a team-mate's misfortune, anger at a refereeing decision, depression about an injury, guilt about cheating. The list of possible emotions in sport is long. Sport without emotion would probably not be sport as we know it.

Emotion defined

Emotions are a psychobiological response to information or events, either real or imagined (recalled or *expected*), that have implications for the immediate or future goals of the person (Beedie et al., 2005; Ekman & Davidson, 1994). Emotions involve numerous brain, nervous, and somatic systems (Damasio, 1998; LeDoux, 1995). Emotions act as a feedback loop between our nervous and endocrine systems and the external (social and physical/environmental) world, which contrasts with mood, which can be conceptualised as an internal (biological) feedback loop (You may already be seeing how emotions – which are driven by real or *expected* events in the social and environmental world – link to placebo responding.) Emotions alter or *bias* many aspects of our conscious mind. For example, when we are anxious, we are more likely to remember moments when we were anxious, more likely to perceive a neutral cue as threatening, more likely to find faults in a proposal and/or be risk-averse in our decision-making about that proposal, and more likely to avoid potentially threatening situations or environments. This is why sports events, job interviews, and presentations to large audiences can be so challenging.

Scientific perspectives on emotion vary (Pace-Schott et al., 2019; Thagard et al., 2021), ranging from social constructionist (Barrett, 2005, 2017) through cognitive/appraisal (Lazarus & Smith, 1988; Moors et al., 2013) to physiological (Damasio & Carvalho, 2013; Damasio, 1998) models. Certainly not all theorists agree on the role of the human body in emotional responses; for example, it has been proposed that emotions are the direct result not of bodily activity but of limbic system *predictions* of body activity (Barrett & Simmons, 2015). There is, however, sufficient aligned evidence from psychology, neuroscience, and biology to support the idea that, in evolutionary and survival terms, emotions function to facilitate a response to the environment, and that response is often physical. To function in this role, emotions modify our biology and physiology, liberating resources and capabilities to facilitate a response to an event. In evolutionary terms, emotional responses often involve movement (fight or flight), the inhibition of movement (fright or freeze), or a strong desire to move also described as an action tendency (Frijda, 1987) which may or may not result in movement but is nonetheless a component of the subjective experience of emotion.

Most emotions are initiated by environmental or psychological events that are sensed, imagined, or recalled in brain regions that communicate via the autonomic nervous and endocrine systems to organs of the body. Resultant biological and physiological responses are fed back to the interoceptive systems of the brain and experienced as feeling (Damasio & Carvalho, 2013). These emotion-induced changes include those below that result from neural-mediated (e.g., adrenaline) and endocrine-mediated (e.g., cortisol) signalling:

- Increased metabolic resources such as oxygen and blood sugar availability (Salovey et al., 2000).
- Modification of resource allocation such as increased blood flow to muscles and reduced blood flow to the viscera (Kreibig, 2010).
- Modification of regulatory processes in anticipation of homeostatic challenges such as increased sweat production and increased threshold for pain sensation (Rhudy & Meagher, 2001).
- Increased mechanical potential for initiating and maintaining movement, such as increased motor cortex activity, motor unit recruitment, and reduced neural inhibition (Lundberg et al., 2002).

Feelings defined

There is an intuitive link between emotions and feelings, but not all feelings are emotions (and, as we'll see, not all emotions are felt). We can feel hungry, which is not an emotion, or angry which is an emotion, and we can feel angry because we're hungry (what has become known as 'hangry') if we perceive that something or someone is stopping us getting the food that will stop us feeling hungry. Other feelings that are not emotions per se but about which we can become emotional include pain, fatigue (although Tim Noakes famously argued that fatigue is in fact an emotion; Noakes, 2012), thirst, and even temperature, in relation to which we are more likely to be angry or anxious when we're very hot or very cold. And as you're aware, pain, fatigue, thirst, and extremes of temperature are all routinely faced by athletes, as is a form of hunger in the need to supplement energy during an event.

There is an almost logical argument that to be called a feeling the thing must be felt, and if it is felt, it is conscious. Pain, fatigue, hunger, thirst, and temperature are indeed all largely conscious processes. Emotions, in contrast, do not have to be conscious, or at least they can affect our physiology and our brain before we are conscious of their presence (perhaps therefore more preconscious than subconscious). In fact, William James, arguably one of the founders of modern psychology, argued that we are not afraid because we have seen a bear; rather, we see the bear because we are afraid. This seemingly counterintuitive argument is supported by research by, among others, James LeDoux who identified that a fear signal can traverse the brain via more than one path, and that the faster of these pathways tends to elude conscious recognition, despite being able to affect our biology. This 'quick and dirty' fear pathway helped our human predecessors, as well as the mammals from whom they evolved and the reptiles before them, to survive in situations in which any deliberate conscious processing of information along the lines "Is that a bear or a shadow?" would have been fatal. Or put another way, individuals who didn't process the presence of a bear (or any other predator) quickly and subliminally were eaten by the bear and didn't pass on to subsequent generations the DNA for their slow-pathway fear responses. Emotions can change very quickly, and we don't always know they're changing until after they've changed.

Interoception defined

The term interoception refers to the brain's receipt and representation of somatic changes, and may or may not enter conscious awareness (Pace-Schott et al., 2019). Interoception is arguably the source of feeling (Attridge, 2019). It is imprecise to allocate interoception to any specific brain region, given that the act of sensing, interpreting, and integrating homeostatic information is related to brain systems involved in attention, detection, discrimination, accuracy, insight, sensibility, and self-report (van der Kolk, 2014). However, there is general agreement that the brain structures involved in interoception include the orbital prefrontal cortex, the medial prefrontal cortex, the somatosensory cortex, the insula, and the anterior and posterior cingulate gyri (Chen et al., 2021; Pollatos et al., 2007; van der Kolk, 2014). In what is an elegant metaphor, the interoceptive signal of ongoing homeostasis has been described as the brain's map of the body's current biological status and resources (Damasio, 2019).

A cognitive account of placebo effects in sport

While a growing body of research locates emotions such as anxiety and depression as targeted outcomes of placebo interventions (Kirsch, 2019), the role of emotions in mediating interventions targeting non-emotion outcomes such as pain or fatigue has received relatively little attention in the published research (Ashar et al., 2017; Flaten et al., 2011; Geers et al., 2021; Wager, 2005). This is understandable; in the context of 'hot' emotions, placebo effects appear relatively cold and cognitive. In fact, when we think of a classic placebo effect in sport we tend to think of a clear process as below:

- Information is conveyed
- Information modifies decision-making
- Modification in decision-making changes outcomes.

For example, a sports nutritionist says to an athlete "I'm about to give you the same supplement that xxxxxxxx uses before competition, and as you know, it has an amazing effect on her performance". This theoretically modifies the expectations of the athlete, possibly from "This is going to be a really hard game" to "I've got an advantage over the opposition" or at least "I will perform better than I originally thought", which in turn might allow the athlete to modify their resource allocation strategy along the lines, "I can commit more resources early on in this game than I would have done if I wasn't taking this supplement". Whether the supplement is real, and capable of influencing performance via the direct biological effects of the supplement, or a placebo, that is incapable of influencing performance via any direct *biological* qualities of the supplement, almost doesn't matter if the athlete has made the decision to commit more resources, especially if doing so will not result in inadequate resources at a later stage of the event. This cognitive account of a placebo effect appears compelling and plays to the idea that athletes have untapped or hidden resources that can be accessed through increased motivational inputs (what we have previously described as 'headroom'; Beedie et al., 2018). In short, it supports the idea that the expectations of the athlete are a significant factor in the placebo effect via direct cognitive mechanisms – information processing, expectation, and decision-making.

And, of course, this is true. But it's also only part of the story. Firstly, because there is no such thing as *pure* cognition. In short, the brain-as-information-processor-model ignores some core processes. Second because even if there were such a thing as pure cognition, those pure cognitions would impact not only on conscious behaviours but also on emotions and biology more generally. That is, the athlete's belief that they now had an advantage would not only impact on their decision-making but also on their emotions. An athlete who was feeling anxious might now be feeling a sense of relief or at least less anxious; an athlete who was feeling agitated might be feeling calmer, an athlete who was feeling depressed might be feeling more hopeful. And those emotions would influence the body of the athlete, potentially exerting a positive effect on the biochemical and physiological processes that are largely responsible for generating and controlling skilled movement.

An emotional account of placebo effects in sport

In 20 years of studying placebo effects among athletes and exercisers, I can make a very binary yet honest statement; not one participant has ever said to me "The placebo capsule you gave me made me *think* differently". However, of those I've asked, a large proportion have used statements that included the words 'feel', 'feeling' or 'felt'. "I felt less anxious", "I felt more up for it", "It felt like the brakes had come off", "I was feeling really energised". Language does not always accurately represent reality, so as a check I think it's fair to point out that I've also delivered cognitive-behavioural interventions to athletes – albeit in narrow contexts such as confidence, decision-making and anxiety regulation – and often been told, for example, "It made me *think* differently". Many, if not most athletes who experience a placebo effect describe it in terms of feeling. This is interesting because many, if not most placebo effects in sport (anecdotally) and in non-sport settings (empirically), are most likely experienced in one of the feelings described above, specifically anxiety, pain, and fatigue.

How does emotion change pain and fatigue?

Pain and fatigue, despite feeling extremely real at the time they are experienced, are both subjective, even illusory processes. Perception of both is affected by many factors, ranging from genetics (Jason et al., 2010; Wang et al., 2017), to personality (Ramírez-Maestre et al., 2004; Stephan et al., 2022), to learning (Apkarian, 2008; Lenaert et al., 2018). Among these factors are emotions. The effect of emotion on perceptions of pain (Rainville et al., 2005) and fatigue (Gibson et al., 2003) have been recognised for a long time. When we are feeling anxious, for example, we are likely to experience pain (Michaelides & Zis, 2019) and fatigue (Jason et al., 2010) as more intense than when we are not feeling anxious.

Research going back almost 30 years has demonstrated the links between anxiety and pain in the context of placebo effects. Benedetti and colleagues administered doses of either proglumide or diazepam to reduce anxiety prior to placebo or nocebo manipulations aimed at modifying the perception of experimentally induced pain. The drugs reduced anxiety and resulted in enhanced placebo analgesia and reduced nocebo hyperalgesia (Benedetti, 1996; Benedetti et al., 1997). And in an interesting reversal of these studies, Benedetti & co-workers (Benedetti et al., 2011) administered the drug pentagastrin, which induces anxiety, panic and fear, to a group of participants and reported that analgesia from a placebo manipulation was reduced.

How do emotions change sports performance?

If emotions such as anxiety modify perceptions of pain and fatigue, and if perceptions of pain and fatigue limit sports performance, a simple causal chain can be seen;

1. Change emotion – reduce anxiety.
2. Change feeling – reduce perception of pain.
3. Change limiting factor – improve performance.

This, however, is a vast oversimplification and as athletes, practitioners, students, and researchers reading this book, you shouldn't simply take my word for it, you should ask "What are the mechanisms?" Different emotions affect performance via different mechanisms, so let's look at the most frequently cited emotion in sport, anxiety, and think about how anxiety changes the body to change performance.

Anxiety and placebo effects in sport

Anxiety is strongly related to fear, and fear prepares the body and brain for a physical response to a real or imagined environmental event. As has been well documented for several decades, anxiety can therefore have a positive effect on sports performance as evidenced in those classic models of performance, such as the Inverted U and multidimensional anxiety theory. While the effects on the body of increasing anxiety might be quite helpful in some contexts – for example, gross movements over short periods of time requiring little cognitive processing or regulation – for many other sport scenarios the increasing physiological arousal and cognitive bias that comes with anxiety is potentially debilitative. Particularly relevant perhaps is the idea that the generalised activation that is associated with anxiety might *interfere* with metabolic and homeostatic processes that are critical to sports performance, especially if that anxiety is of a high intensity for a significant period ahead of performance; put simply, anxiety is a survival mechanism and, like most such processes, comes with high costs in metabolic processes such as blood glucose and oxygen, in turn, increasing the energy cost of movement in neuromuscular processes such as the coordinated activation and relaxation of antagonistic muscles (not only reducing the quality of movement but also further increasing the energy cost of movement), and in cognitive processes such as concentration and decision-making, rendering the economic and strategic regulation of the resources of the body more problematic. And in some respects, sport performance is all about the successful deployment of metabolic, cognitive, and emotional resources.

As is proposed in numerous models of anxiety and performance, there is a 'sweet spot' between a level at which the anxiety is sufficiently low to have no positive effect on performance and sufficiently high to have a negative effect. The intensity of anxiety in question varies between athletes, and sometimes between contexts (an athlete might prefer lower levels of anxiety before a final than before a heat), and finding this sweet spot is important for performance. With this in mind, researchers, practitioners and athletes have proposed and tested numerous strategies, many of which work for many people, some of which work only for a few, and some of which were ultimately ineffective. Arguably, however, any intervention that can predictably and reliably position an athlete's anxiety in the sweet spot is legitimately described as an emotion regulation strategy, because that is what it has done, regulated an emotion to a specific and facilitative place. And as was the case with Judy in the vignette at the start of this chapter, one such intervention is to modify an athlete's *expectations* of their performance, which is often the root cause of the anxiety in the first place.

How do expectations change emotions?

In the scenario at the beginning of the chapter, Judy's expectations are causing anxiety. Her coach does not address the anxiety directly by using, for example, imagery or self-talk but does so by modifying the expectations that are causing the anxiety. If he had instead said "I've just heard that your opponent broke the World record in the qualifying round" he would have, unhelpfully, changed her expectations in the opposite direction and potentially increased the anxiety (or created a nocebo effect, see below). Either way, the point is expectations will almost certainly have an effect on emotion, so changes in expectations likewise change emotions. And emotions change performance.

Are placebo interventions therefore simply a sub-category of emotion regulation?

If reduced anxiety can reduce perceptions of pain and fatigue and thereby enhance sports performance, and if placebo-induced expectations can reduce anxiety, are placebo interventions in fact little more than deceptive emotion regulation interventions? Emotion regulation has received a substantial degree of attention in both research (Gross & Thompson, 2007) and applied contexts (Lane et al., 2012). Emotion regulation in sport can take many forms, ranging from the traditional such as pre-performance routines, imagery, self-talk, bio-feedback, various forms of physical rituals (warm-up, progressive muscular relaxation, regulated breathing) and music, through to the athlete isolating themselves, even the use of supplements, medicines, and complementary & alternative treatments. In fact, many apparently strategies might be as much about regulating emotions as about any argued-for direct or biological effects associated with them (see the chapter by Beedie on complementary medicine in this book).

What about the nocebo effect in sport?

So, a placebo intervention can be a form of emotion regulation intervention. Let's consider the following ideas: Athletes expect to experience negative emotions and feelings, they expect anxiety which is a prototypical emotion as well as pain and fatigue which are both feelings that themselves promote emotions. Given that anxiety, pain, and fatigue are highly placebo-responsive, sport is a placebo-rich environment. But for the same reason, sport is also a nocebo-rich environment with anxiety, pain and fatigue all being highly nocebo-responsive. If positive effects of reducing anxiety, pain, and fatigue be described as a placebo effect, then any cue that increases any of these – for example, negative expectations of an event – could be described as a nocebo. This is an idea that warrants further research (see also Chapter 2).

Summary

Placebo effects appear to be cognitive things, but, like emotions, they have a significant affective component. Through modifying expectations and thereby modifying emotions, placebo interventions can bring about changes in performance-limiting feelings such as pain and fatigue in sport, as well as health variables beyond sport such as pain, fatigue, immune function, anxiety and depression. In fact, given that pain and fatigue have been found to be highly placebo-responsive, sport can be considered a placebo-rich environment. By the same token, sport is also a nocebo-rich environment with pain and fatigue all being highly responsive to *negative expectations* and to the emotional consequences of those.

Placebo interventions can be used to modify emotion and are therefore legitimately described as emotion regulation. As suggested above, emotion regulation has attracted substantial attention in sport (Lane et al., 2012), in many respects in response to the significant database of research attesting to the role of affect more broadly in sports performance, from Morgan's Mental Health model in the 1970s (Morgan, 1974), to the refinement of mood performance models by Peter Terry (Terry, 1995) and Andy Lane (Lane et al., 2001), the extension of Morgan's work into overtraining syndrome by Jack Raglin and others (Raglin & Wilson, 2000), to the idiographic emotional zones proposed by Juri Hanin (Hanin, 2000) and the challenging of existing ideas of emotion with respect to fatigue by Noakes (Noakes, 2012) and both the associated central governor model (Noakes et al., 2001) and its extension, the integrative governor theory by Alan St Clair-Gibson and colleagues (St Clair Gibson et al., 2018).

The study of emotion and placebo effects in sport is valuable for what both teach us about the mind, the brain, and the bodies of athletes. It is important never to forget that cognition, emotion, and action all take place within an integrated system. While reduction and analysis are important processes of science, it is important to consider how each piece contributes to the whole. Future research should therefore consider questions such as the following:

1. Whether a change in emotional status is a necessary, if not sufficient component of a placebo effect?
2. Which emotions might mediate the outcomes of placebo interventions on performance-limiting factors such as pain or fatigue?
3. Whether an athlete's pre-intervention mood state can facilitate or inhibit a placebo effect?
4. Which existing emotion regulation interventions of phenomena might be wholly or partly effective via changes in expectation (for example, directional anxiety; Jones & Hanton, 2001)?

References

Apkarian, A. V. (2008). Pain perception in relation to emotional learning. *Current Opinion in Neurobiology, 18*(4), 464–468. https://doi.org/10.1016/j.conb.2008.09.012

Ashar, Y. K., Chang, L. J., & Wager, T. D. (2017). Brain mechanisms of the placebo effect: An affective appraisal account. *Annual Review of Clinical Psychology, 13*, 73–98.

Attridge, M. (2019). A Global Perspective on Promoting Workplace Mental Health and the Role of Employee Assistance Programs. *American Journal of Health Promotion, 33*(4), 622–629. https://doi.org/10.1177/0890117119838101c

Barrett, L. F. (2005). Feeling is perceiving: Core affect and conceptualization in the experience of emotion. In *Emotion and consciousness.* (pp. 255–284). The Guilford Press. https://doi.org/10.1016/j.tics.2007.01.005

Barrett, L. F. (2017). Categories and their role in the science of emotion. *Psychological Inquiry, 28*(1), 20–26. https://doi.org/10.1080/1047840X.2017.1261581

Barrett, L. F., & Simmons, W. K. (2015). Interoceptive predictions in the brain. *Nature Reviews Neuroscience, 16*(7), 419–429. https://doi.org/10.1038/nrn3950

Beedie, C., Benedetti, F., Barbiani, D., Camerone, E., Cohen, E., Coleman, D., Davis, A., Elsworth-Edelsten, C., Flowers, E., Foad, A., & Harvey, S. (2018). Consensus statement on placebo effects in sports and exercise: The need for conceptual clarity, methodological rigour, and the elucidation of neurobiological mechanisms. *European Journal of Sport Science, 18*(10), pp. 1383–1389.

Beedie, C., Terry, P., & Lane, A. (2005). Distinctions between emotion and mood. *Cognition & Emotion, 19*(6), 847–878. https://doi.org/10.1080/02699930541000057

Beedie, C. J., & Foad, A. J. (2009). The placebo effect in sports performance: A brief review. *Sports Medicine, 39*, 313–329.

Benedetti, F. (1996). The opposite effects of the opiate antagonist naloxone and the cholecystokinin antagonist proglumide on placebo analgesia. *Pain, 64*(3). https://journals.lww.com/pain/Fulltext/1996/03000/The_opposite_effects_of_the_opiate_antagonist.17.aspx

Benedetti, F., Amanzio, M., Casadio, C., Oliaro, A., & Maggi, G. (1997). Blockade of nocebo hyperalgesia by the cholecystokinin antagonist proglumide. *Pain, 71*(2), 135–140.

Benedetti, F., Amanzio, M., & Thoen, W. (2011). Disruption of opioid-induced placebo responses by activation of cholecystokinin type-2 receptors. *Psychopharmacology, 213*, 791–797.

Chen, W. G., Schloesser, D., Arensdorf, A. M., Simmons, J. M., Cui, C., Valentino, R., Gnadt, J. W., Nielsen, L., Hillaire-Clarke, C. S., Spruance, V., Horowitz, T. S., Vallejo, Y. F., & Langevin, H. M. (2021). The Emerging Science of Interoception: Sensing, Integrating, Interpreting, and Regulating Signals within the Self. *Trends in Neurosciences, 44*(1), 3–16. https://doi.org/10.1016/j.tins.2020.10.007

Damasio, A. (2019). *The Strange Order of Things: Life Feeling and the Making of Cultures.* Pantheon Books.

Damasio, A., & Carvalho, G. B. (2013). The nature of feelings: Evolutionary and neurobiological origins. *Nature Reviews Neuroscience, 14*(2), 143–152. https://doi.org/10.1038/nrn3403

Damasio, A. R. (1998). Emotion in the perspective of an integrated nervous system. *Brain Research Reviews, 26*(2), 83–86. https://doi.org/10.1016/S0165-0173(97)00064-7

Davis, A. J., Hettinga, F., & Beedie, C. (2020). You don't need to administer a placebo to elicit a placebo effect: Social factors trigger neurobiological pathways to enhance sports performance. *European Journal of Sport Science, 20*(3), 302–312.

Ekman, P. E., & Davidson, R. J. (1994). *The nature of emotion: Fundamental questions.* Oxford University Press.

Flaten, M. A., Aslaksen, P. M., Lyby, P. S., & Bjørkedal, E. (2011). The relation of emotions to placebo responses. *Philosophical Transactions of the Royal Society B: Biological Sciences, 366*(1572), 1818–1827. https://doi.org/10.1098/rstb.2010.0407

Frijda, N. H. (1987). Emotion, cognitive structure, and action tendency. *Cognition and Emotion, 1*(2), 115–143. https://doi.org/10.1080/02699938708408043

Geers, A. L., Faasse, K., Guevarra, D. A., Clemens, K. S., Helfer, S. G., & Colagiuri, B. (2021). Affect and emotions in placebo and nocebo effects: What do we know so far? *Social and Personality Psychology Compass, 15*(1), e12575. https://doi.org/10.1111/spc3.12575

Gibson, A. S. C., Baden, D. A., Lambert, M. I., Lambert, E. V., Harley, Y. X. R., Hampson, D., Russell, V. A., & Noakes, T. D. (2003). The Conscious Perception of the Sensation of Fatigue. *Sports Medicine, 33*(3), 167–176. https://doi.org/10.2165/00007256-200333030-00001

Gross, J. J., & Thompson, R. A. (2007). Emotion regulation: Conceptual foundations. In *Handbook of emotion regulation* (pp. 3–24). Guilford Press.

Hanin, Y. L. (2000). Individual Zones of Optimal Functioning (IZOF) Model: Emotion-performance relationship in sport. In *Emotions in sport* (pp. 65–89). Human Kinetics.

Hurst, P., Schipof-Godart, L., Szabo, A., Raglin, J., Hettinga, F., Roelands, B., Lane, A., Foad, A., Coleman, D., & Beedie, C. (2020). The placebo and nocebo effect on sports performance: A systematic review. *European Journal of Sport Science, 20*(3), 279–292.

Jason, L. A., Evans, M., Brown, M., & Porter, N. (2010). What is Fatigue? Pathological and Nonpathological Fatigue. *PM&R, 2*(5), 327–331. https://doi.org/10.1016/j.pmrj.2010.03.028

Jones, G., & Hanton, S. (2001). Pre-competitive feeling states and directional anxiety interpretations. *Journal of Sports Sciences, 19*(6), 385–395. https://doi.org/10.1080/026404101300149348

Kirsch, I. (2019). Placebo effect in the treatment of depression and anxiety. *Frontiers in Psychiatry, 10*. https://www.frontiersin.org/articles/10.3389/fpsyt.2019.00407

Kreibig, S. D. (2010). Autonomic nervous system activity in emotion: A review. *Biological Psychology, 84*(3), 394–421. https://doi.org/10.1016/j.biopsycho.2010.03.010

Lane, A. M., Beedie, C. J., Jones, M. V., Uphill, M., & Devonport, T. J. (2012). The BASES Expert Statement on emotion regulation in sport. *Journal of Sports Sciences, 30*(11), 1189–1195. https://doi.org/10.1080/02640414.2012.693621

Lane, A. M., Terry, P. C., Beedie, C. J., Curry, D. A., & Clark, N. (2001). Mood and performance: Test of a conceptual model with a focus on depressed mood. *Psychology of Sport and Exercise, 2*(3), 157–172. http://dx.doi.org/10.1016/S1469-0292(01)00007-3

Lazarus, R. S., & Smith, C. A. (1988). Knowledge and appraisal in the cognition—emotion relationship. *Cognition & Emotion, 2*(4), 281–300. https://doi.org/10.1080/02699938808412701

LeDoux, J. E. (1995). Emotion: Clues from the Brain. *Annual Review of Psychology, 46*(1), 209–235. https://doi.org/10.1146/annurev.ps.46.020195.001233

Lenaert, B., Boddez, Y., Vlaeyen, J. W. S., & van Heugten, C. M. (2018). Learning to feel tired: A learning trajectory towards chronic fatigue. *Behaviour Research and Therapy, 100*, 54–66. https://doi.org/10.1016/j.brat.2017.11.004

Lieberman, M. D. (2006). Social cognitive neuroscience: A review of core processes. *Annual Review of Psychology*, *58*(1), 259–289. https://doi.org/10.1146/annurev. psych.58.110405.085654

Lundberg, U., Forsman, M., Zachau, G., Eklöf, M., Palmerud, G., Melin, B., & Kadefors, R. (2002). Effects of experimentally induced mental and physical stress on motor unit recruitment in the trapezius muscle. *Work & Stress*, *16*(2), 166–178. https://doi.org/10.1080/02678370210136699

Michaelides, A., & Zis, P. (2019). Depression, anxiety and acute pain: Links and management challenges. *Postgraduate Medicine*, *131*(7), 438–444. https://doi.org/10. 1080/00325481.2019.1663705

Moors, A., Ellsworth, P. C., Scherer, K. R., & Frijda, N. H. (2013). Appraisal theories of emotion: State of the art and future development. *Emotion Review*, *5*(2), 119–124. https://doi.org/10.1177/1754073912468165

Morgan, W. P. (1974). Selected psychological considerations in sport. *Research Quarterly. American Alliance for Health, Physical Education and Recreation*, *45*(4), 374–390. https://doi.org/10.1080/10671315.1974.10615285

Noakes, T. (2012). Fatigue is a brain-derived emotion that regulates the exercise behavior to ensure the protection of whole body homeostasis. *Frontiers in Physiology*, *3*. https://doi.org/10.3389/fphys.2012.00082

Noakes, T. D., Peltonen, J. E., & Rusko, H. K. (2001). Evidence that a central governor regulates exercise performance during acute hypoxia and hyperoxia. *Journal of Experimental Biology*, *204*(18), 3225–3234. 10.1242/jeb.204.18.3225

Pace-Schott, E. F., Amole, M. C., Aue, T., Balconi, M., Bylsma, L. M., Critchley, H., Demaree, H. A., Friedman, B. H., Gooding, A. E. K., Gosseries, O., Jovanovic, T., Kirby, L. A. J., Kozlowska, K., Laureys, S., Lowe, L., Magee, K., Marin, M.-F., Merner, A. R., Robinson, J. L., Smith, R. C., Spangler, D. P., Van Overveld, M., & VanElzakker, M. B. (2019). Physiological feelings. *Neuroscience & Biobehavioral Reviews*, *103*, 267–304. https://doi.org/10.1016/j.neubiorev.2019.05.002

Pollatos, O., Schandry, R., Auer, D. P., & Kaufmann, C. (2007). Brain structures mediating cardiovascular arousal and interoceptive awareness. *Brain Research*, *1141*, 178–187. https://doi.org/10.1016/j.brainres.2007.01.026

Raglin, J. S., & Wilson, G. S. (2000). Overtraining in athletes. *Emotions in sport*, *191207*, 506.

Rainville, P., Bao, Q. V. H., & Chrétien, P. (2005). Pain-related emotions modulate experimental pain perception and autonomic responses. *Pain*, *118*(3), 306–318. https://doi.org/10.1016/j.pain.2005.08.022

Ramírez-Maestre, C., Martínez, A. E. L., & Zarazaga, R. E. (2004). Personality characteristics as differential variables of the pain experience. *Journal of Behavioral Medicine*, *27*(2), 147–165. https://doi.org/10.1023/B:JOBM.0000019849. 21524.70

Rhudy, J. L., & Meagher, M. W. (2001). The role of emotion in pain modulation. *Current Opinion in Psychiatry*, *14*(3), 241–245. https://doi.org/10.1097/ 00001504-200105000-00012

Salovey, P., Rothman, A. J., Detweiler, J. B., & Steward, W. T. (2000). Emotional states and physical health. *American Psychologist*, *55*(1), 110. https://doi.org/10.1037/ 0003-066X.55.1.110

St Clair Gibson, A., Swart, J., & Tucker, R. (2018). The interaction of psychological and physiological homeostatic drives and role of general control principles in the regulation of physiological systems, exercise and the fatigue process – The integrative governor theory. *European Journal of Sport Science, 18*(1), 25–36. https://doi.org/10.1080/17461391.2017.1321688

Stephan, Y., Sutin, A. R., Luchetti, M., Canada, B., & Terracciano, A. (2022). Personality and fatigue: Meta-analysis of seven prospective studies. *Scientific Reports, 12*(1), 9156. https://doi.org/10.1038/s41598-022-12707-2

Terry, P. (1995). The efficacy of mood state profiling with elite performers: A review and synthesis. *The Sport Psychologist, 9*(3), 309–324. https://doi.org/10.1123/tsp.9.3.309

Thagard, P., Larocque, L., & Kajić, I. (2021). Emotional change: Neural mechanisms based on semantic pointers. *Emotion.* https://doi.org/10.1037/emo0000981

van der Kolk, B. A. (2014). *The body keeps the score: Brain, mind, and body in the healing of trauma.* Viking.

Wager, T. D. (2005). Expectations and anxiety as mediators of placebo effects in pain. *Pain, 115*(3). https://journals.lww.com/pain/Fulltext/2005/06000/Expectations_and_anxiety_as_mediators_of_placebo.1.aspx

Wang, T., Yin, J., Miller, A. H., & Xiao, C. (2017). A systematic review of the association between fatigue and genetic polymorphisms. *Brain, Behavior, and Immunity, 62*, 230–244. https://doi.org/10.1016/j.bbi.2017.01.007

7

ARE PLACEBO EFFECTS A PERCEPTUAL ILLUSION?

Placebo effects on performance within the Bayesian brain

Aaron Greenhouse-Tucknott, Jake B. Butterworth, James G. Wrightson, and Jeanne Dekerle

Introduction

Widespread interest in placebo effects and nocebo effects exists within multiple and diverse scientific disciplines as it provides a window into the powerful interactions between brain and body (Wager & Atlas, 2015). As outlined already in previous chapters of this book, in sport there is an increasing appreciation that placebo effects can provide invaluable insight into factors that determine performance (Beedie & Foad, 2009; Hurst et al., 2020). Yet despite this interest, mechanisms of placebo effects are unclear. This has resulted in the formulation of several theories which focus on understanding its principle psychological underpinnings (Peiris et al., 2018).

Progress in our appreciation of how the brain works has concomitantly offered new scope for understanding the placebo mechanisms. The classic view of our brains was one of a passive *stimulus–response* organ, where our perception of the world and how we interact with it (i.e., our actions) is almost exclusively defined by the sensory signals our brains receive (e.g., we feel pain because peripheral nociceptors are activated signalling potential tissue damage). However, contemporary perspectives propose that our brains are, in fact, actively engaged in constructing our own view of the world through inferential processes. That is, our brains use prior (learned or acquired) expectancies to form predictions and infer the cause-and-effect relationships underlying the sensations we experience. This enables us to anticipate and, most importantly, understand the conditions of the external (i.e., outside world) and internal (i.e., the body) environment from the multiple, noisy, and ultimately uncertain streams of sensory inputs that our brains have to contend with (Clark, 2013; Friston, 2009; Hohwy, 2016). Through this

DOI: 10.4324/9781003229001-7

inferential process, our perception of the world may be generated, and our actions guided.

Within cognitive neuroscience, computational models of brain function based on the concepts of the *Bayesian brain* and *predictive processing* – which will be expanded upon below – are gaining recognition as potential explanations of placebo mechanisms (Büchel et al., 2014; Geuter et al., 2017; Ongaro & Kaptchuk, 2019; Petzschner et al., 2017). These accounts can also help us understand how our brains predictively control the internal conditions of our bodies during exercise, influencing exercise regulation and consequently physical performance (Greenhouse-Tucknott et al., 2021). Combined, they may therefore help us to understand the causes and impact of placebo effects in sport and exercise. The present chapter will attempt to provide a brief introduction to these models, and describe the current evidence supporting their application within placebo-based research (i.e., the study of placebo hypoalgesia), before concluding with an evaluation of the possible implications for the study of placebo effects in sport and exercise.

The Bayesian brain hypothesis: Navigating our uncertain world based on prior expectations

The Bayesian brain hypothesis (Knill & Pouget, 2004; Ongaro & Kaptchuk, 2019) offers a descriptive account of how the brain combines sensory inputs with prior knowledge to deal with the inherent uncertainty present within the sensory information our brains receive. The basic premise is that we combine new information with existing knowledge in a (approximately) statistically optimal way, in line with Thomas Bayes' famous probabilistic theorem (for an introduction see: Knill & Pouget, 2004; O'Reilly et al., 2012). Through evolutionary processes and our personal encounters with the world, we learn and assign probabilities to the values of sensory stimuli (both internal and external) to which we are exposed. When we are presented with a particular sensory stimulus, our experience can be based on an integration of our initial expectations of it and the sensory data received. The statistically optimal 'compromise' between our initial expectations and the encountered sensory evidence reflects the (conditional) probability our initial expectations were correct given the evidence (this is referred to as *posterior* in Bayesian terminology; Figure 7.1). In the Bayesian brain, construction and maintenance of an internal (*generative*) model of the world enables us to formulate hypotheses about sensory states which are essentially 'hidden' from the brain, accessible only indirectly through our senses (Friston, 2012). When presented with sensory inputs, our model of the world provides us with an ability to infer the most likely cause of these states, enabling us to form perceptions and directing our actions.

Underlying its Bayesian formulation, prior expectations and the likelihood of incoming sensory inputs are represented probabilistically in our brains

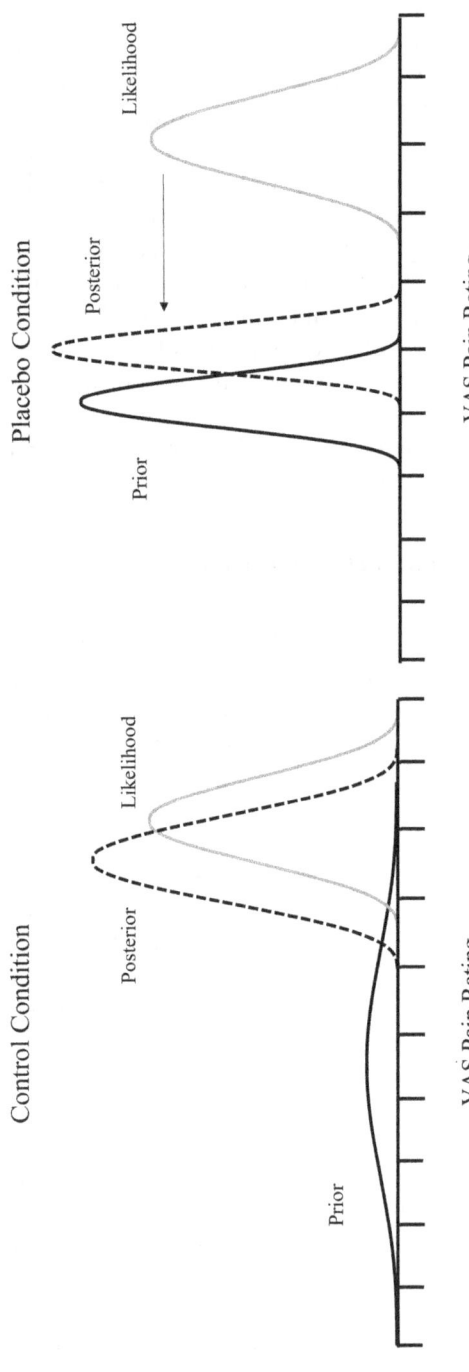

FIGURE 7.1 The foundation of generative models of the world following Bayes' theorem. Our perceptions and actions (i.e. the posterior) represents the statistically optimal combination of the probability of our prior predictions of sensory states and the likelihood of the sensory data. Probability distributions in the figure are depicted as Gaussian or normal distributions. The precision of these estimates can be visualised as the width of the probability distributions (see insert on the left of the diagram). If the sensory evidence that we receive is strong and precise, deviating away from our initial predictions, we may be forced to update our models to better represent the world around us. That is, our posterior may be shifted away from our prior predictions closer to the sensory evidence (i.e. likelihood). Conversely, if we believe that the sensory evidence is likely to be unreliable (i.e. lower precision), our perception may conform closer to our modelled predictions (i.e. prior). In predictive processing, the difference between our prior predictions of sensory states and the likelihood of those states generates a measure of the accuracy of our predictions, the prediction error. The prediction error is communicated to other levels within the hierarchically structured system containing our model of the world and used in the comparison between predictions at that level.

(Figure 7.1). That is, they are not represented by a single value, but the probability of a particular value occurring (Knill & Pouget, 2004). By utilising probability, our brain can deal with the uncertain sensory information it receives by both appreciating and accounting for it. This is achieved by using a precision-weighting when combining prior expectations with the sensory evidence. Precision broadly reflects the reliability of our prior expectations and the incoming sensory data (Friston, 2009; Kanai et al., 2015), determining their relative influence in forming perception and driving action. If predictions are imbued with higher precision than the sensory data, then our perceptions and actions will be heavily influenced by our model's predictions of what *should* be, possibly at the expense of the actual information received. Conversely, if our predictions are afforded lower precision than the sensory data, the latter will be heeded to, which will cause our model's predictions to be updated and fall in line with the sensory information the brain has gathered. For example, imagine playing Rugby on a foggy morning. When defending, the perception of the opponent's position may be driven to a greater extent by previous experiences, and the reliability afforded to the sensory evidence (i.e., visual information) may be reduced given the conditions. Precision is itself predicted, thus subject to the same inferential processes, ultimately defining both perception and action. It is believed to be encoded, in part, by the action of neuromodulators, including dopamine (Friston et al., 2012) and possibly endogenous opioids (Büchel et al., 2014), which may provide some links to mechanisms of placebo effects (see Chapter 4).

Predictive processing broadly refers to a neurobiologically plausible scheme (Shipp, 2016) used in the implementation of Bayesian inference (Friston, 2005; Rao & Ballard, 1999). (For a glossary of terms, see Table 7.1.) Essentially, the theory proposes that our model's predictions and any arising prediction error – that is, the part of the sensory data that is not compatible with our predictions (i.e., the mismatch) – flow between levels of a hierarchically structured system within the brain, which represents our model of the world. Fundamentally, prediction error is at the core of this theory. Our brains are believed to be in the game of prediction error minimisation (Hohwy, 2016). By minimising prediction error our brains can optimise our model of the world (Friston, 2010). Optimisation is vital, as our brains' primary goal is the maintenance of a small set of predictable states across our lifespan, broadly analogous to the maintenance of homeostasis (Friston, 2010). This is, however, a particularly complicated task for the brain to maintain, and it is not a linear process. Indeed, there may be situations where short-term prediction error may be tolerated if it allows us to gain knowledge that can be used to minimise prediction error over the long term (Schwartenbeck et al., 2013). Nevertheless, prediction error can be minimised in two different ways: First, prediction error may be used to update the predictions generated by our model of the world to fit with the sensory information received. This represents a fundamental

TABLE 7.1 Glossary of terms used within predictive processing

Term	Definition / description
Active inference	An extension of inference through predictive processes to include action. Prediction error can be minimised through action and selective sampling to ensure that the sensory data matches initial predictions.
Bayesian brain hypothesis	The idea that the brain uses probabilistic (generative) models of the world to optimally integrate prior knowledge and sensory evidence, in (approximate) accordance to Bayesian theory. Enables (statistical) inference through minimisation of the divergence between prior knowledge and sensory evidence (e.g., prediction error).
Generative model	An internal representation that models how sensory signals are generated from hidden causes. It is called generative as it can be used to generate mock sensory signals given an estimate of the hidden cause.
Hidden states	Environmental conditions and causes of sensory stimuli that cannot be directly observed, so must be inferred.
Hierarchy	The structure of the organisation of predictors, which accounts for their operation on different spatio-temporal scales.
Likelihood	A probability distribution representing how the prior is related to any new information gathered. Comparison of the prior and the likelihood results in a difference measure (i.e., prediction error).
Perception	In predictive processing, corresponds to the inversion of generative models of sensory inputs, so that hidden causes or states can be mapped from the sensory inputs received.
Posterior	A probability distribution based on the statistically optimal combination of a prior and a likelihood.
Precision	Mathematically, the inverse of the variance of a variable. A precise variable is one that is seen as reliable. Low precision reflects low reliability. Precision enables us to factor in the degree of uncertainty in our predictions and the sensory evidence.
Prediction	A representation of a likely future state of the organism and/or its environment.
Predictive error	The difference, or mismatch, between a measurement or actual state, and the predictive estimate of that state.
Predictive processing	A broad term used to describe a theory of cognition and perception that is realised through the passing of predictions and prediction error between levels of a neural hierarchy.
Prior	A probability distribution of the causes of data, representing the believed causes before the data has been observed.
Probability distribution	A mathematical function that provides the probabilities of the occurrence of different possible outcomes.

feature of both perceptual inference and learning. Second, prediction error can be minimised by making sure that sensory data fits with what is predicted through actions (Friston, 2009). That is, through action we can make sure we selectively sample the sensory inputs that match our model's predictions. This is the basis of *active inference* (Adams et al., 2013), which essentially argues that perception and action represent a unified process within prediction error minimisation.

Placebo effects and the Bayesian brain: Current evidence

Under the Bayesian brain hypothesis, placebo effects have been described as a *perceptual illusion* (Anchisi & Zanon, 2015). It is proposed that the precision of our predictions is central to understanding this phenomenon (Büchel et al., 2014). The basic premise is thus: placebo treatments work by generating very strong (i.e., highly precise) predictions about the outcome of a treatment, such that our predictions dominate over sensory evidence during their integration. The strongest placebo effects should therefore be seen when both the benefit and reliability (i.e., precision) of a treatment are predicted to be high (Figure 7.2). However, when precision is lower (e.g., when the outcome of the treatment is less certain), or if sensory information is afforded greater salience (e.g., in the case of large prediction errors because predicted states are too far removed from reality), then placebo effects may be attenuated or even lost.

The idea that uncertainty (i.e., precision) plays an important role in placebo effects has long been acknowledged. For example, altering patients' expectations of the effectiveness of a purported analgesic treatment through verbal instruction has been shown to influence the magnitude of placebo-induced hypoalgesia, with the greatest effect seen when patients were most certain about the efficacy of the treatment (Pollo et al., 2001). However, it is only recently that research has sought to establish whether the response to uncertainty in placebo effects conforms to the Bayesian formulation proposed under predictive processing (Anchisi & Zanon, 2015; Grahl et al., 2018; Jung et al., 2017). This research has focussed exclusively on the study of pain ratings and placebo-hypoalgesia. Anchisi and Zanon (2015) demonstrated that a Bayesian approach could explain placebo-associated pain relief. In this study, participants were briefed that they would receive a treatment (i.e., transcutaneous electrical nerve stimulation [TENS]) that would reduce the experience of the pain evoked by electrical stimulation of the foot. To foster positive expectations of the effectiveness of the treatment, the authors associated the application of the treatment to a visual cue presented on a computer, with participants told that the treatment was active when the cue was coloured green and inactive when coloured red. Surreptitiously, during an initial conditioning phase of the

Prior: How probable was the hypothesis before observing the evidence?

Likelihood: How probable is the evidence given the hypothesis is true?

Posterior: How probable is the hypothesis given the observed evidence?

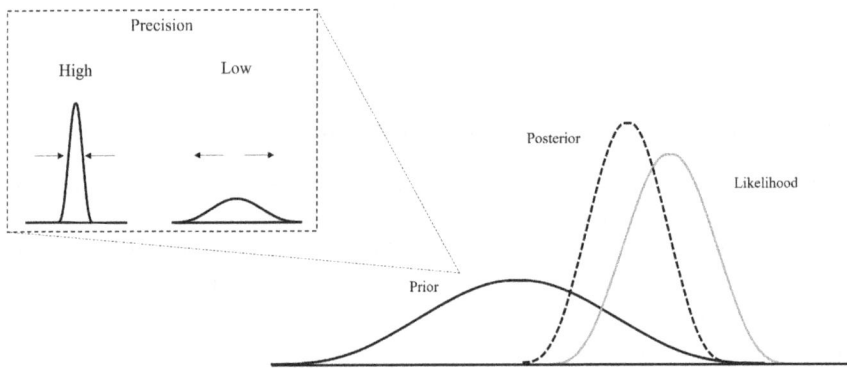

FIGURE 7.2   The proposed effect of placebo on pain ratings based on Bayesian theory. The prior distribution represents our predictions, the likelihood represents the incoming sensory data, and the posterior represents the integration of the two. In the control condition, an uncertain (i.e. imprecise) expectation about pain may be generated, with the probability distribution shallow and flat. Consequently, our perception of a painful stimulus (i.e. the posterior) will likely conform closer, if not exactly to the incoming sensory data. Under the placebo condition, however, we may hold a strong and precise prediction that the treatment will cause us to experience a low level of pain. This prior may be more precise than the sensory data, such that is causes our perception of pain (i.e. the posterior) to be shifted closer to our prior predictions. Figure is adapted from Büchel et al. (2014).

experiment, the authors reduced the intensity of the electrical stimulation when participants expected the treatment to be working (i.e., when the visual cue was green), such that they experienced less pain when they believed treatment to be active. During the test phase of the placebo effect, the painful stimuli was not manipulated, remaining at a constant intensity, but participants were shown the same visual cues such that they believed the treatment had been 'applied'. The authors constructed a Bayesian model to describe participants' pain ratings and noted that it was supported by substantial evidence based on participants' responses. In summary, pain ratings could be effectively modelled based on the rules of Bayesian probabilistic reasoning (Anchisi & Zanon, 2015).

Providing more specific insight into the importance of precision within this computation, Grahl et al. (2018) manipulated individuals' expected efficacy of a sham analgesic treatment (again, pain relief through TENS). Expectations were once more set by altering the intensity of a painful stimulus (in this study, a contact heat stimulator placed on participants' forearms) during a conditioning period. Individuals in the high-precision group were led to believe that the treatment would evoke consistent and effective pain relief, whereas those in the low-precision group were led to experience the treatment as more variable in reducing pain, therefore forming an expectation that the benefit of the treatment was more uncertain. Again, during the test phase of the placebo effect, participants were exposed to an identical noxious temperature. Behaviourally, the authors reported a greater placebo effect on ratings of pain in the high-precision group. A Bayesian-based model applied to individual responses, which incorporated the precision of prior expectations in the calculations, outperformed control models in explaining the subjective pain responses. This suggested that individuals affording greater precision to positive predictions of the effectiveness of the treatment experienced the largest placebo effect on pain ratings (Grahl et al., 2018). Though firm conclusions must be tempered by the limited models with which the Bayesian models were compared, the results do suggest that a Bayesian integration of expectations and sensory evidence, sensitive to the precision of those variables, can be used to understand placebo effects such as placebo-induced hypoalgesia, at a perceptual level.

Placebos, predictions, and physical performance: A proposal

The evidence described above indicates that placebo effects, such as placebo-induced hypoalgesia, can effectively be described by viewing our brain as a statistical machine engaged in Bayesian inference. By changing predictions generated from our model of the world, under placebo conditions, our perceptions (and actions) are influenced to a greater extent by what we hypothesise the world to be like. This is thought to be due to the level of precision afforded to outcome-based predictions, which may be so high that our model does not properly consider the sensory evidence (Schenk et al., 2017) – essentially ignoring it or explaining it away. The emerging support for this computational account may therefore allow us to better understand placebo-induced changes found within sport and exercise settings.

Our perceptions of, and feelings about, the demands placed on us during physical tasks holds a vital role in our ability to persist in such tasks (Greenhouse-Tucknott et al., 2020). Placebo interventions have been shown to alter our perceptions of physical work, typically alleviating how hard or difficult a physical task is perceived to be (Mothes et al., 2017; Pollo et al., 2008). The strength and precision of our predictions under placebo conditions may be such that prediction errors arising from data obtained from our bodies and the external environment may be attenuated, thus exerting limited influence on our perception of how effortful the task is (Kuppuswamy, 2017). Not limited to just placebos, perceptual responses evoked by all ergogenic aids may be highly dependent upon our predictions of their effects. For example, it was recently shown that a reduction in individuals' perceived exertion during exercise coupled with caffeine supplementation could be reversed and actually increased when participants believe that the caffeine they had ingested was in fact a detrimental lactic acid capsule (Azevedo et al., 2021). This supports the idea that what we perceive is contextualised by our predictions of the world which, if the prediction is strong and precise enough, can be disassociated from the sensory evidence obtained (e.g., physiological states). The outlined account offers a computationally tractable way to understand how this may come to pass.

As stated, prediction error can be minimised in two ways by appealing to both perceptual learning and action. Action does not just reflect our overt behaviour (e.g., a pacing strategy during a race or the ending of a time to task failure), but also incorporates autonomic functions used to control physiologic processes (Barrett & Simmons, 2015). We will just focus on the former here for ease of presentation. Under placebo conditions, positive, precise predictions generated by a purported intervention may see us to push ourselves harder in order to match our prior expectations. Indeed, when athletes were falsely informed that they had taken caffeine and were made aware of its beneficial effects for performance, they were shown to pace a 1000-m run differently to control conditions, going out harder and faster during the first 400 m only (Hurst et al., 2019). However, if our actions conform to our predictions, then why do the athletes only run faster during the initial 400 m? Why does the placebo effect wane? Under the Bayesian proposal, this may be attributed to a progressive greater precision-weighting afforded to prediction error (and, conversely, lesser precision-weighing afforded to predictions). The consequence of running faster may be that it incurs larger, less predictable changes in our physiological state over time. To maintain predicted sensory states, the athletes may inevitably have to slow down (Hurst et al., 2019) as a way of attenuating this increasingly salient prediction error. Active inference therefore provides a base to understand interactions between perceptions and action and how both may be modulated by placebo interventions within sporting contexts.

Central to the proposal is the idea of precision. Though we lack direct evidence to appropriately interrogate this idea in reference to sporting performance, we find conceptual support of its influence in the literature. This may also allow us to offer a mechanism to a pertinent question: who is susceptible to placebo effects? Hurst and colleagues demonstrated that the effect of placebo (i.e., an undetermined potent supplement) on repeated sprints was variable between individuals, with no group effect observed as a result (Hurst et al., 2017). Investigating who within the sample was most susceptible to placebo effects, the authors identified that a beneficial effect on performance was only seen in participants who expressed intentions to take ergogenic supplements (Beedie et al., 2020). If we assume that intention to use, in part, reflects a strong belief in the reliability of the effectiveness of supplementation in pursuit of a desired outcome, then the results appeal to the proposition that greater precision afforded to positive predictions of a purported intervention may see actions dictated by a dominance of predictions under placebo conditions. Interestingly, beneficial performance effects evoked by placebos in sport settings appear to be greater when the purported intervention is a banned ergogenic aid (i.e., doping substances; Hurst et al., 2020). This is possibly because the headlines and exposure these substances receive provides us with a very clear (i.e., precise) expectation of their effectiveness (Hurst et al., 2020). As such, the precision we afford to the predicted outcomes of taking such substances may be greater than other substances or interventions in which the effect is less certain.

The described account offers clearly testable hypotheses (Büchel et al., 2014). Accordingly, examination of whether the combination of predictions and sensory evidence, conforming to Bayesian principles, can explain altered physical performance under placebo conditions is now required. Perhaps one of the most pertinent applications of the outlined account of placebo effects within a sporting context may be in understanding the consequences for fatigue. Fatigue is proposed to be the common currency underlying all research investigating placebo effects within physical performance (Beedie et al., 2020). Predictive processing accounts have offered a new appreciation of the possible computational development of fatigue (Greenhouse-Tucknott et al., 2021; Stephan et al., 2016). Persistent detection of a mismatch between what we predict our sensory states to be and sensory evidence we receive (i.e., prediction error) may see us lose confidence in our models' ability to predict the world around us (Greenhouse-Tucknott et al., 2021; Stephan et al., 2016). Bayesian approaches describe this as the basis of our conscious experience of fatigue, which may accompany a change in behaviour, favouring rest as we try and restore self-efficacy in our predictions. Endowing our predictions with greater precision, limiting the detection and/or impact of prediction error, placebos may provide important insight into this proposal, as they offset the development of fatigue. Placebo-based interventions may thus provide invaluable insight into the new proposals outlining how computations performed by the brain lead to the development of fatigue.

Conclusions

The only way our brain can understand and direct behaviour within the world outside of our head is to predict and infer the sensory inputs it receives. Introducing the theory of predictive processing, we have described a computational approach, based on Bayesian theory, that may be used to understand the emergence of placebo effects within our brains. Here, expectations arising from placebo treatments ultimately shifts the balance in the way the brain deals with sensory uncertain towards a reliance on prior beliefs, which may have concomitant effects on resource allocation and therefore on performance. This framework may help us better understand why we run faster, push harder and fatigue slower, when exposed to the powerful influence of placebos.

References

Adams, R. A., Shipp, S., & Friston, K. J. (2013). Predictions not commands: Active inference in the motor system. *Brain Structure and Function*, *218*, 611–643.

Anchisi, D., & Zanon, M. (2015). A Bayesian perspective on sensory and cognitive integration in pain perception and placebo analgesia. *PloS one*, *10*(2), e0117270.

Azevedo, P. H., Oliveira, M. G., Tanaka, K., Pereira, P. E., Esteves, G., & Tenan, M. S. (2021). Perceived exertion and performance modulation: Effects of caffeine ingestion and subject expectation. *The Journal of Sports Medicine and Physical Fitness*, *61*(9), 1185–1192.

Barrett, L. F., & Simmons, W. K. (2015). Interoceptive predictions in the brain. *Nature Reviews Neuroscience*, *16*(7), 419–429. https://doi.org/10.1038/nrn3950

Beedie, C., Benedetti, F., Barbiani, D., Camerone, E., Lindheimer, J., & Roelands, B. (2020). Incorporating methods and findings from neuroscience to better understand placebo and nocebo effects in sport. *European Journal of Sport Science*, *20*(3), 313–325.

Beedie, C. J., & Foad, A. J. (2009). The placebo effect in sports performance: A brief review. *Sports Medicine*, *39*, 313–329.

Büchel, C., Geuter, S., Sprenger, C., & Eippert, F. (2014). Placebo analgesia: A predictive coding perspective. *Neuron*, *81*(6), 1223–1239.

Clark, A. (2013). Whatever next? Predictive brains, situated agents, and the future of cognitive science. *Behavioral and Brain Sciences*, *36*(3), 181–204.

Friston, K. (2005). A theory of cortical responses. *Philosophical Transactions of the Royal Society B: Biological Sciences*, *360*(1456), 815–836.

Friston, K. (2009). The free-energy principle: A rough guide to the brain? *Trends in Cognitive Sciences*, *13*(7), 293–301.

Friston, K. (2010). The free-energy principle: A unified brain theory? *Nature Reviews Neuroscience*, *11*(2), 127–138.

Friston, K. (2012). The history of the future of the Bayesian brain. *Neuroimage*, *62*(2), 1230–1233.

Friston, K. J., Shiner, T., FitzGerald, T., Galea, J. M., Adams, R., Brown, H., Dolan, R. J., Moran, R., Stephan, K. E., & Bestmann, S. (2012). Dopamine, affordance and active inference. *PLoS Computational Biology*, *8*(1), e1002327.

Geuter, S., Koban, L., & Wager, T. D. (2017). The cognitive neuroscience of placebo effects: Concepts, predictions, and physiology. *Annual Review of Neuroscience*, *40*, 167–188.

Grahl, A., Onat, S., & Büchel, C. (2018). The periaqueductal gray and Bayesian integration in placebo analgesia. *Elife*, *7*, e32930.

Greenhouse-Tucknott, A., Butterworth, J., Wrightson, J. G., Smeeton, N. J., Critchley, H., Dekerle, J., & Harrison, N. A. (2021). Toward the unity of pathological and exertional fatigue: A predictive processing model. *Cognitive, Affective, & Behavioral Neuroscience*, 1–14.

Greenhouse-Tucknott, A., Wrightson, J. G., Raynsford, M., Harrison, N., & Dekerle, J. (2020). Interactions between perceptions of fatigue, effort, and affect decrease knee extensor endurance performance following upper body motor activity, independent of changes in neuromuscular function. *Psychophysiology*, 57(9), e13602.

Hohwy, J. (2016). The self-evidencing brain. *Noûs*, 50(2), 259–285.

Hurst, P., Foad, A., Coleman, D., & Beedie, C. (2017). Athletes intending to use sports supplements are more likely to respond to a placebo. *Medicine & Science in Sports & Exercise (MSSE)*.

Hurst, P., Schipof-Godart, L., Hettinga, F., Roelands, B., & Beedie, C. (2019). Improved 1000-m running performance and pacing strategy with caffeine and placebo: A balanced placebo design study. *International Journal of Sports Physiology and Performance*, 15(4), 483–488.

Hurst, P., Schipof-Godart, L., Szabo, A., Raglin, J., Hettinga, F., Roelands, B., Lane, A., Foad, A., Coleman, D., & Beedie, C. (2020). The placebo and nocebo effect on sports performance: A systematic review. *European Journal of Sport Science*, 20(3), 279–292.

Jung, W.-M., Lee, Y.-S., Wallraven, C., & Chae, Y. (2017). Bayesian prediction of placebo analgesia in an instrumental learning model. *PloS One*, 12(2), e0172609.

Kanai, R., Komura, Y., Shipp, S., & Friston, K. (2015). Cerebral hierarchies: Predictive processing, precision and the pulvinar. *Philosophical Transactions of the Royal Society B: Biological Sciences*, 370(1668), 20140169.

Knill, D. C., & Pouget, A. (2004). The Bayesian brain: The role of uncertainty in neural coding and computation. *Trends in Neurosciences*, 27(12), 712–719. https://doi.org/10.1016/j.tins.2004.10.007

Kuppuswamy, A. (2017). The fatigue conundrum. *Brain*, 140(8), 2240–2245.

Mothes, H., Leukel, C., Seelig, H., & Fuchs, R. (2017). Do placebo expectations influence perceived exertion during physical exercise? *PloS one*, 12(6), e0180434.

O'Reilly, J. X., Jbabdi, S., & Behrens, T. E. (2012). How can a Bayesian approach inform neuroscience? *European Journal of Neuroscience*, 35(7), 1169–1179.

Ongaro, G., & Kaptchuk, T. J. (2019). Symptom perception, placebo effects, and the Bayesian brain. *Pain*, 160(1). https://journals.lww.com/pain/Fulltext/2019/01000/Symptom_perception,_placebo_effects,_and_the.1.aspx

Peiris, N., Blasini, M., Wright, T., & Colloca, L. (2018). The placebo phenomenon: A narrow focus on psychological models. *Perspectives in Biology and Medicine*, 61(3), 388.

Petzschner, F. H., Weber, L. A., Gard, T., & Stephan, K. E. (2017). Computational psychosomatics and computational psychiatry: Toward a joint framework for differential diagnosis. *Biological Psychiatry*, 82(6), 421–430.

Pollo, A., Amanzio, M., Arslanian, A., Casadio, C., Maggi, G., & Benedetti, F. (2001). Response expectancies in placebo analgesia and their clinical relevance. *Pain*, 93(1), 77–84.

Pollo, A., Carlino, E., & Benedetti, F. (2008). The top-down influence of ergogenic placebos on muscle work and fatigue. *European Journal of Neuroscience*, 28(2), 379–388.

Rao, R. P., & Ballard, D. H. (1999). Predictive coding in the visual cortex: A functional interpretation of some extra-classical receptive-field effects. *Nature Neuroscience*, 2(1), 79–87.

Schenk, L. A., Sprenger, C., Onat, S., Colloca, L., & Büchel, C. (2017). Suppression of striatal prediction errors by the prefrontal cortex in placebo hypoalgesia. *Journal of Neuroscience*, *37*(40), 9715–9723.

Schwartenbeck, P., FitzGerald, T., Dolan, R., & Friston, K. (2013). Exploration, novelty, surprise, and free energy minimization. *Frontiers in Psychology*, *4*, 710.

Shipp, S. (2016). Neural elements for predictive coding. *Frontiers in Psychology*, *7*, 1792.

Stephan, K. E., Manjaly, Z. M., Mathys, C. D., Weber, L. A., Paliwal, S., Gard, T., Tittgemeyer, M., Fleming, S. M., Haker, H., & Seth, A. K. (2016). Allostatic self-efficacy: A metacognitive theory of dyshomeostasis-induced fatigue and depression. *Frontiers in Human Neuroscience*, *10*, 550.

Wager, T. D., & Atlas, L. Y. (2015). The neuroscience of placebo effects: Connecting context, learning and health. *Nature Reviews Neuroscience*, *16*(7), 403–418.

8

CAN WE REPLACE OXYGEN, AT LEAST PARTIALLY, WITH A PLACEBO?

Placebo effects at high altitude

Fabrizio Benedetti

Introduction

What has emerged over recent years is that the magnitude of placebo effects varies across different conditions, from small to large, for example in pain, both experimental and clinical, in motor disorders, especially Parkinson's disease, behavioural conditioning of the immune and endocrine system, some psychiatric conditions such as depression and anxiety, as well as physical performance in sport (Benedetti, 2020; Hurst et al., 2019). It is now clear that placebos activate mechanisms similar to those activated by drugs. For example, there is compelling experimental evidence that placebos can modulate the same receptors that are modulated by narcotics and cannabinoids (Benedetti et al., 2011; Petrovic et al., 2002). Similarly, placebos can activate dopamine receptors, which are the very same as those activated by dopaminergic anti-Parkinson drugs (de la Fuente-Fernández et al., 2002; De La Fuente-Fernandez & Stoessl, 2002) and can modulate the cyclooxygenase pathway in the same way as non-steroid anti-inflammatory drugs (Benedetti & Dogue, 2015; Benedetti et al., 2015; Benedetti et al., 2014). To better understand placebo effects across a variety of conditions, oxygen-dependent physiological functions, such as ventilation, are particularly interesting for several reasons. In fact, they give rise to challenging and provocative questions such as: Can we replace oxygen, at least partially, with a placebo? The aim of this chapter is to present experimental evidence that this is really possible, namely, that oxygen can be partially replaced by a placebo (fake oxygen) with little change, if any, in the overall functioning of the body.

DOI: 10.4324/9781003229001-8

Oxygen-dependent physiological functions

Ventilation, oxygenation, circulation and perfusion are considered the four most important critical life functions. Oxygen is at the core of all of these functions. It goes from atmospheric air to the lungs, it is exchanged with carbon dioxide in the lungs and spreads to the blood stream, to then reach all the peripheral tissues and cells, e.g. the brain and neurons. When little oxygen is available in the air, a condition called hypoxia, several body functions counterbalance the oxygen shortage by triggering at least three fundamental compensatory responses: an increase in ventilation (hyperventilation) through the activation of chemoreceptors; an increase in circulation through increased cardiac output, e.g. heart rate increase; and an increase in perfusion through vasodilation, e.g. cerebral vasodilation, whereby prostaglandins (PG) such as PGE2 have been found to be involved (Benedetti & Dogue, 2015).

One crucial question is to understand whether placebo effects occur for any physiological function in which oxygen is involved. It goes without saying that this poses several ethical problems in the clinical setting, because we would need to study patients in hypoxic conditions, namely, with low blood oxygen saturation (SO2). For example, replacing even a tiny amount of oxygen with a placebo in a patient with either respiratory failure or admitted to an intensive care unit would certainly be unethical, and investigating the effects of placebo treatments on SO2 or impaired ventilation would be unfeasible at the bedside. Therefore, what is needed in order to study placebo effects in oxygen-dependent functions is a model that is both ethical and amenable to scientific investigation.

High altitude

A natural model of hypoxia is represented by high altitude: as altitude increases, oxygen decreases. What is important is not so much oxygen concentration but rather oxygen partial pressure. As altitude increases, oxygen pressure decreases. For example, oxygen pressure at sea level is 159 mmHg, whereas it drops to 102 mmHg at 3500 m. Mountain medicine indicates three altitude regions that reflect the lowered amount of oxygen in the atmosphere: high altitude (1500–3500 m), very high altitude (3500–5500 m), and extreme altitude (above 5500 m; International Society for Mountain Medicine, 2017). On the basis of the way our body responds to oxygen shortage, high altitude can be subdivided into four zones of adaptation or acclimatisation (Schmidt & Thews, 1989) (Figure 8.1), although several other subdivisions do exist. The zone from the sea level to about 1800–2000 m is called "indifferent", as there are no appreciable effects on the body, at least in most people. The zone from 2000 m to about 4000 m is called "full compensation zone", as many physiological responses compensate the low oxygen pressure, e.g. hyperventilation,

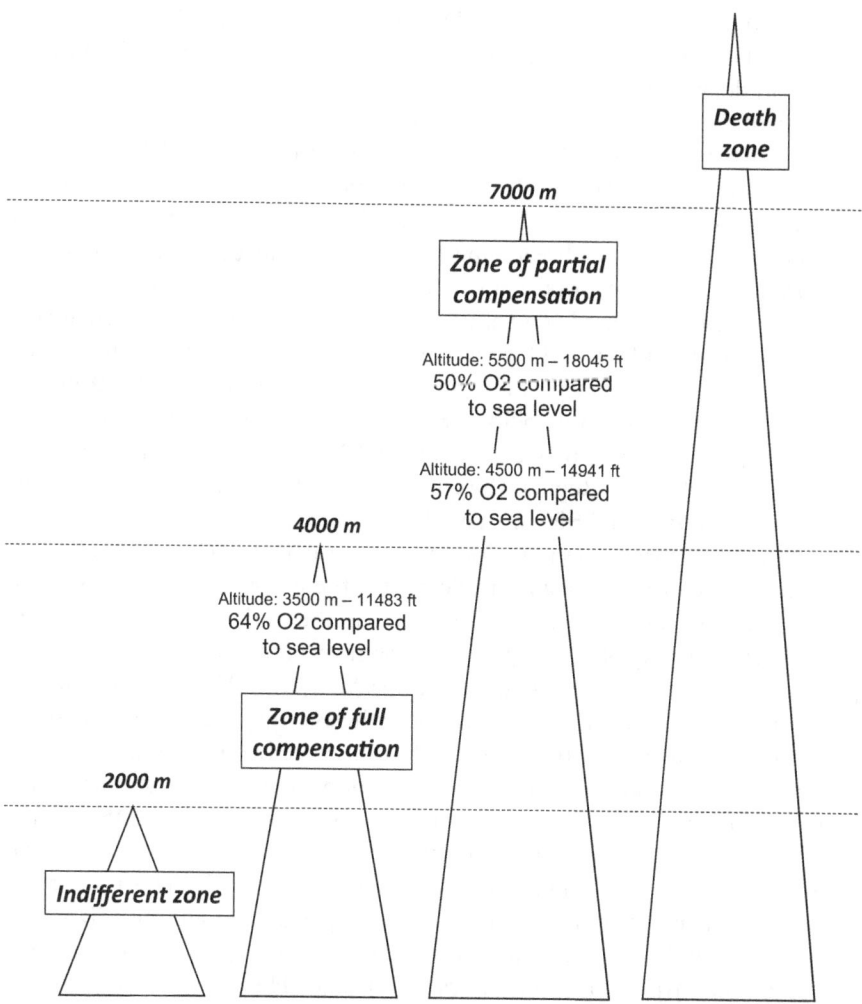

FIGURE 8.1 General subdivision of different altitude zones, and the altitudes where we have data about placebo effects (3500 m, 4500 m, 5500 m).

increased heart rate, cerebral vasodilation. The zone from 4000 m to about 7000 m is called "partial compensation zone", as many physiological responses are not capable of compensating for oxygen shortage. Here, many severe symptoms can develop, such as pulmonary oedema and cerebral oedema, which can result in severe permanent damage and even death. The zone above about 7000 m is called "death zone": most people die at this altitude, as the amount of oxygen is insufficient to sustain human life and the body is incapable of acclimatising. The concept of the *death zone* (originally the *lethal zone*) was first conceived in 1953 by Edouard Wyss-Dunant, a Swiss doctor, in an article about acclimatisation (Wyss-Dunant, 1953). Although this is a very general subdivision and description (Figure 8.1), it gives a general idea of the high-altitude model of hypoxia.

Most of the studies on the placebo effects at high altitude have been performed in the zone of full compensation, where oxygen availability is 64% compared to sea level (Figure 8.1). The reason for that is simple: we need a degree of hypoxia in which several physiological compensatory responses develop, yet they are not threatening for life. This is made possible by one of the locations where we work, namely, the Center for Hypoxia at the Plateau Rosà Laboratories, located at an altitude of 3500 m in the Matterhorn area at the border between Italy and Switzerland. Only a couple of studies have been performed in the zone of partial compensation, at altitudes of 4500 m and 5500 m, where oxygen availability is 57% and 50%, respectively, compared to the sea level (Figure 8.1; Benedetti et al., 2018). The studies at 4500 m have been performed at the Regina Margherita Hut on the Monte Rosa in Italy, whereas the studies at 5500 m have been done at the Simon Bolivar and Cristobal Colon twin peaks in Colombia and at the Denali (former McKinley) mountain in Alaska. The main problem with these very high altitudes is the small number of subjects who can participate in the study, which is justified by the inherent difficulty of bringing healthy volunteers to high altitude. For example, only 6 subjects were tested at the Regina Margherita Hut, 5 at the Denali, and 4 at the Colombian twin peaks. Nonetheless, they have provided some important information on the placebo effect in severe hypoxic conditions.

The clinical condition triggered by hypobaric (low oxygen pressure) hypoxia at high altitude is known as acute mountain sickness (AMS) (Imray et al., 2010; Wilson et al., 2009), which is usually diagnosed by means of the Lake Louise Score (LLS) questionnaire (Sutton et al., 1992). This is aimed at detecting several symptoms, such as headache, nausea/vomiting, dizziness, insomnia, as well as neurological symptoms, which emphasise the complex nature of this hypoxia-related clinical syndrome. Headache is the cardinal symptom, and indeed the most common symptom even at relatively low altitudes. Headache is also one of the most studied symptoms of AMS, although the details of its pathophysiology are partly unknown. As far as we know, there are at least two pathways triggering high-altitude headache. The first is represented by the acute effects of hypoxia on PG synthesis through the cyclooxygenase (COX) enzyme, with the formation of PGD2, PGF2, PGE2, PGI2 (prostacyclin), and thromboxane (TX) A2 (Benedetti et al., 2014; Richalet et al., 1991). One of the most important effects of these eicosanoids, particularly PGE2, is represented by vasodilation, which is thought to be the principal factor inducing acute hypoxia headache (Busse et al., 1984; Fredricks et al., 1994; Messina et al., 1992; Ray et al., 2002), although the direct stimulation of nociceptive afferents cannot be ruled out (Kawabata, 2011). However, a second pathway that is important for high-altitude headache is represented by the hypoxia-related hyperventilation that, in turn, induces the excessive elimi-nation of carbon dioxide (CO_2) with the consequent increase in blood pH (alkalosis; West, 2005). To support the important role of alkalosis in AMS and high-altitude headache is the therapeutic effect of blood pH reduction by means of acetazolamide (Leaf & Goldfarb, 2007). Besides the reduction of alkalosis with acetazolamide, there are at least two other effective treatments for high-altitude headache: oxygen inhalation (Bärtsch et al., 1990; Benedetti & Dogue, 2015) and oral cyclooxygenase inhibitors, such as aspirin (Benedetti et al., 2014; Burtscher et al., 1998). Whereas the former restores blood oxy-gen saturation (SO2), thus decreasing hyperventilation and alkalosis, the latter inhibits the hypoxia-activated cyclooxygenase and PG synthesis, thus reducing cerebral vasodilation (Benedetti et al., 2015).

Replacing oxygen with placebo

There is today experimental evidence that placebos can mimic the effects of oxygen for oxygen reductions up to 50% compared to the sea level. Most of the evidence comes from studies at 3500 m (64% oxygen compared to sea level), 4500 m (57% oxygen), and 5500 m (50% oxygen) (Benedetti et al., 2018), as well as from high-altitude simulations in the lab at the sea level (Torres-Peralta et al., 2016). These studies show that placebos can affect oxygen-dependent functions like ventilation, circulation, perfusion, as well as overall performance, but not oxygenation. Figure 8.2 shows the experimental condition at high altitude, where different physiological recordings have been carried out.

Oxygenation

In no case was a change in SO2 found after placebo administration (see the studies described below and Figure 8.3), which indicates that placebos cannot in any way affect blood oxygenation. This is not surprising, as blood oxygen-ation is due to the direct diffusion of oxygen from the lungs to the blood stream, without any involvement of the central nervous system. Indeed, it is unlikely that a placebo can change the way oxygen diffuses from air to blood. As will be discussed in detail below, this is one of the most interesting findings of all these studies, because it shows that placebos may affect many body func-tions without any change in oxygen content of the body.

Ventilation

A hypoventilation effect can be elicited by a placebo after oxygen precondi-tioning. In fact, the typical compensatory hyperventilation of high altitude can be inhibited by administering oxygen and this can be mimicked by placebo.

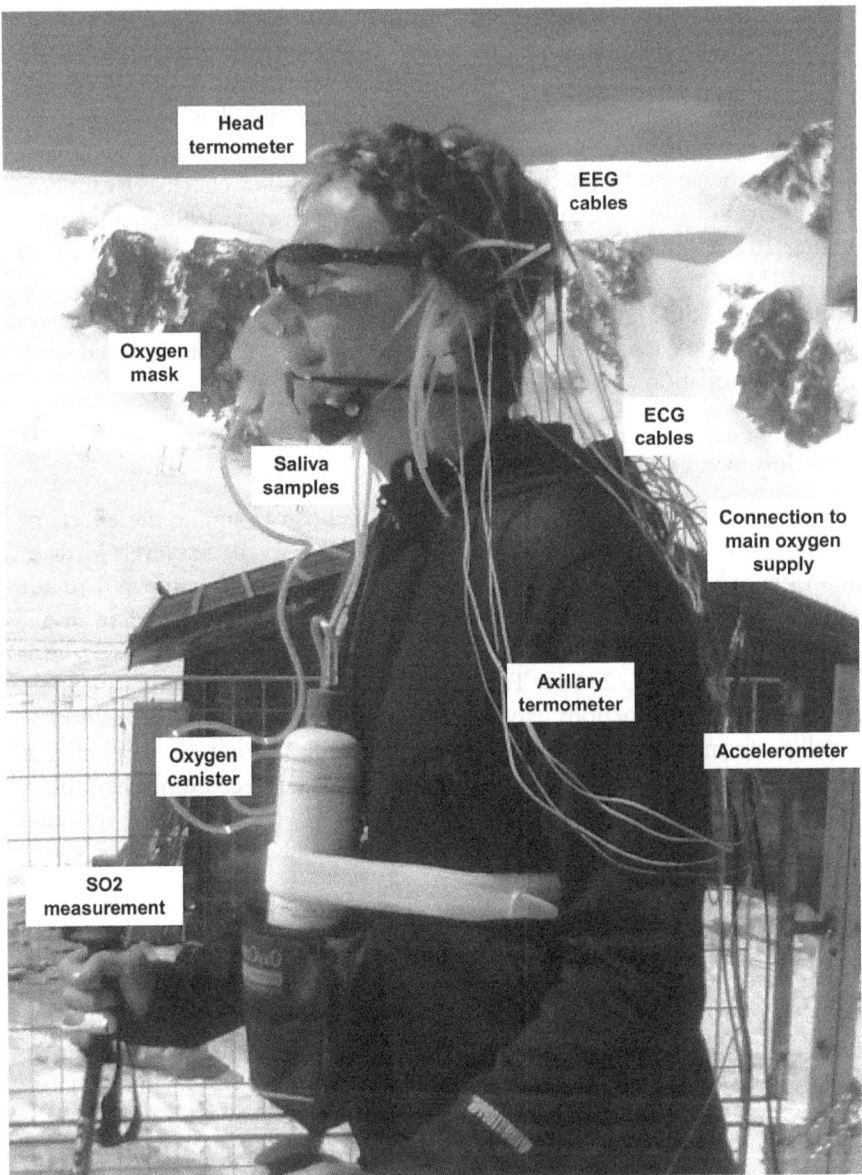

FIGURE 8.2 Four physiological functions (ventilation, oxygenation, circulation, perfusion), along with physical performance, have been investigated by recording several physiological parameters.

It can be seen in Figure 8.3 that, whereas placebo given for the first time does not produce any effect on minute ventilation (Vmin), expressed as litres/min, a placebo after prior oxygen exposure for n times induces substantial changes of Vmin. This effect is present with 64% oxygen at 3500 m (Figure 8.3;

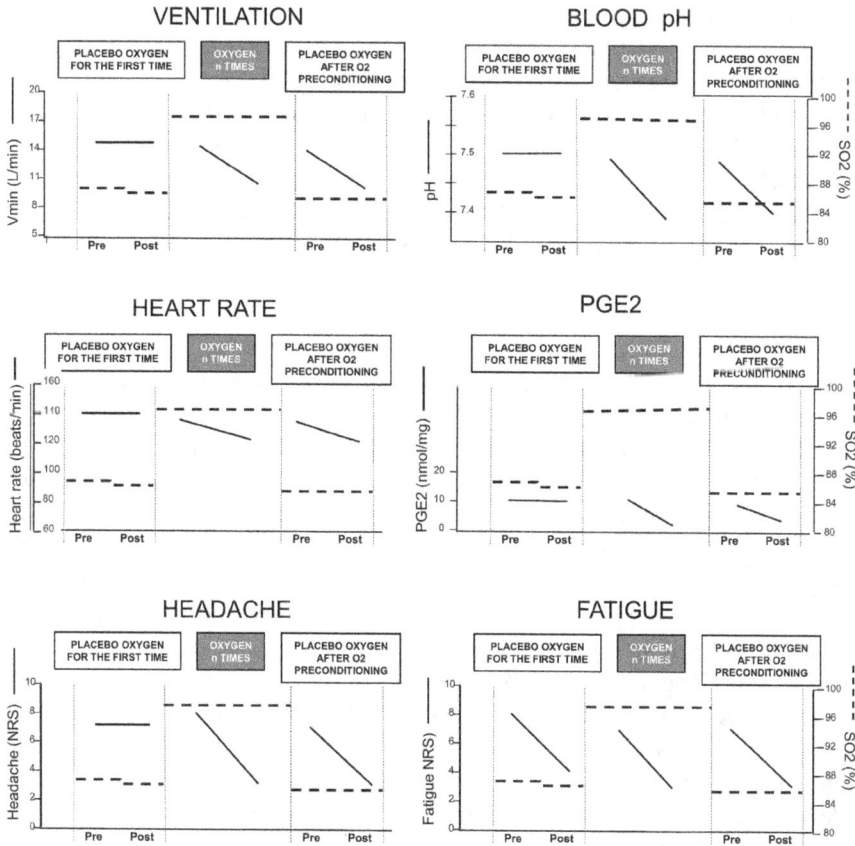

FIGURE 8.3 The effects of placebo given for the first time, of oxygen, and of placebo after oxygen preconditioning on minute ventilation, blood pH, heart rate, PGE2, headache, fatigue at 3500 m. Note that there no changes in SO2 after placebo administration. Also note that fatigue is the only placebo-responsive parameter that does not require oxygen preconditioning. Same effects occur at 4500 m 5500 m.

Benedetti et al., 2015), as well as with 57% oxygen at the Regina Margherita Hut and 50% oxygen at the Denali and Colombian twin peaks (Benedetti et al., 2018). Two important points need to be emphasised. First, oxygen preconditioning is crucial for a placebo respiratory effect to occur (Benedetti et al., 2015), thus the placebo respiratory effect is basically a conditioned hypoventilation response. Second, this effect on ventilation can be seen with an oxygen reduction up to 50%.

The effects on ventilation by placebo are quite important, as they are not limited to ventilation itself, but extend to blood pH. In fact, hyperventilation at high altitude is accompanied by an increase in blood pH (alkalosis). Oxygen decreases both hyperventilation and blood pH. Likewise, placebo after oxygen preconditioning can produce the very same effect, namely, a decrease in both hyperventilation and blood pH (Figure 8.3). This effect is present even at 5500 m, where oxygen is 50% compared to sea level. Therefore, placebos may affect both ventilation and its consequences on blood pH. It is crucial to note in Figure 8.3 that, not surprisingly, SO2 increases after oxygen administration. Conversely, no change in SO2 occurs after placebo administration, which indicates that hypoventilation and pH responses are not due to SO2 *per se*, but rather to a SO2-independent learning mechanism.

Circulation

As for ventilation, a similar bradycardic effect can be elicited by a placebo after oxygen preconditioning. In fact, the typical compensatory tachycardia of high altitude can be inhibited by administering oxygen, and this effect can be mimicked by placebo. In Figure 8.3, it can be seen that, whereas placebo given for the first time does not produce any effect on heart rate, expressed as beats/min, a placebo given after prior oxygen exposure for n times induces substantial changes in heart rate. This effect is present with 64% (3500 m), 57% (4500 m) and 50% (5500 m) oxygen compared to sea level. Therefore, as with ventilation, oxygen preconditioning is crucial for a placebo bradycardic response to occur (Benedetti & Dogue, 2015). We can thus consider the placebo bradycardic effect as a conditioned bradycardic response. Most interestingly, this effect on heart activity can be seen with an oxygen reduction up to 50%. Again, note in Figure 8.3 that whereas SO2 increases after oxygen administration, no change in SO2 occurs after placebo administration, which indicates that bradycardia is not due to SO2 *per se*, but rather to a SO2-independent learning mechanism.

Perfusion

The experimental evidence that placebos may affect cerebral perfusion through vasodilation is indirect, as no direct measurement of cerebral blood flow has been performed so far. Evidence comes from the assessment of some biomarkers that are known to be involved in cerebral vasodilation. In particular, PGE2 is known to induce vasodilation, a typical compensatory response to high-altitude hypoxia, and is thought to be the principal factor inducing acute hypoxia headache (Busse et al., 1984; Fredricks et al., 1994; Messina et al., 1992; Ray et al., 2002). Therefore, headache is the clinical expression of cerebral vasodilation, which represents an interesting parameter to assess in order to understand the effects of PGE2 on cerebral blood vessels.

As for ventilation and heart rate at high altitude, a similar reduction in PGE2 can be elicited by a placebo after oxygen preconditioning. The typical PGE2 increase at high altitude can be blocked by administering oxygen and this effect can be mimicked by placebo. Figure 8.3 shows that whereas a placebo given for the first time does not produce any effect on PGE2, a placebo given after prior oxygen exposure for n times induces a substantial decrease in PGE2. Again, this effect is present with 64%, 57% and 50% oxygen compared to sea level. Therefore, as for ventilation and heart rate, oxygen preconditioning is crucial for a placebo PGE2 reduction to occur (Benedetti et al., 2015). Thus, this placebo effect is basically a conditioned PGE2 response. It is worth noting that this effect on heart activity can be seen with an oxygen reduction up to 50%.

In the same way as PGE2 can be considered an indirect measure of cerebral vasodilation, so a headache can be considered the clinical expression of cerebral vasodilation. It can be seen in Figure 8.3 that placebos can reduce a headache only after oxygen preconditioning, thus supporting the findings for PGE2. It is important to note that two types of headache have been tested: at rest and after exercise. Only post-exercise headache has been found to be affected by placebos, however; no effect was observed for headache at rest. Once more, it can be seen in Figure 8.3 that whereas SO2 increases after oxygen administration, no change in SO2 occurs after placebo administration, which indicates that PGE2 modulation and post-exercise headache are not due to SO2 *per se*, but rather to a SO2-independent learning mechanism.

Performance

Overall performance in hypoxic conditions is reduced because of the changes in ventilation, heart activity and perfusion of different organs, including brain and muscles. However, what is emerging today is that SO2 is not completely responsible for overall performance, at least within some limits, central nervous system mechanisms, including complex psychological factors, playing an important role. These factors are related to the so-called "central command" or "central governor", a mechanism implying that several physiological parameters, like heart rate, arterial blood pressure, pulmonary ventilation, and muscle performance, could be altered by manipulating the subject's perception of exercise (Krogh & Lindhard, 1913). Placebos have been proposed to impact on this central governor of fatigue. The output of this centre would continuously regulate exercise performance to avoid reaching maximal physiological capacity. This would provide protection against damage on one hand, and constant availability of a reserve capacity on the other (Noakes et al., 2005; St Clair Gibson et al., 2003). Placebos could then represent a psychological means to signal to the central governor to release the brake, allowing an increase in performance. Muscle fatigue has also been found to be affected by a central governor (Noakes et al., 2005; St Clair Gibson et al., 2003; St Clair Gibson et al., 2006). In many studies, athletes are usually asked to perform at their limit, and placebos apparently act by pushing this limit forward (Piedimonte et al., 2015). To support this perspective, many studies suggest that fatigue and overall performance are of central rather than peripheral origin.

As can be seen in Figure 8.3, fatigue is the only parameter that does not require oxygen preconditioning in order to be sensitive to placebos (Benedetti et al., 2018). In other words, differently from the above-mentioned conditions, a placebo given for the first time, along with positive verbal suggestions of fatigue reduction and performance improvement, is sufficient to reduce fatigue. The effect of placebo alone, without any oxygen preconditioning, is so powerful that it is also present with an oxygen reduction of 50% compared to sea level. It is crucial to note that this effect on fatigue is independent of SO2, thus supporting the central command model of perceived fatigue and performance.

The perceived fatigue has a powerful influence on overall performance. Benedetti et al. (2018) showed that the time to complete 3000 steps with a stepper worsened from sea level to high altitude, and that performance returned to that of sea level following administration of both oxygen and placebo (Figure 8.4). Importantly, placebo was given without any oxygen preconditioning, and this

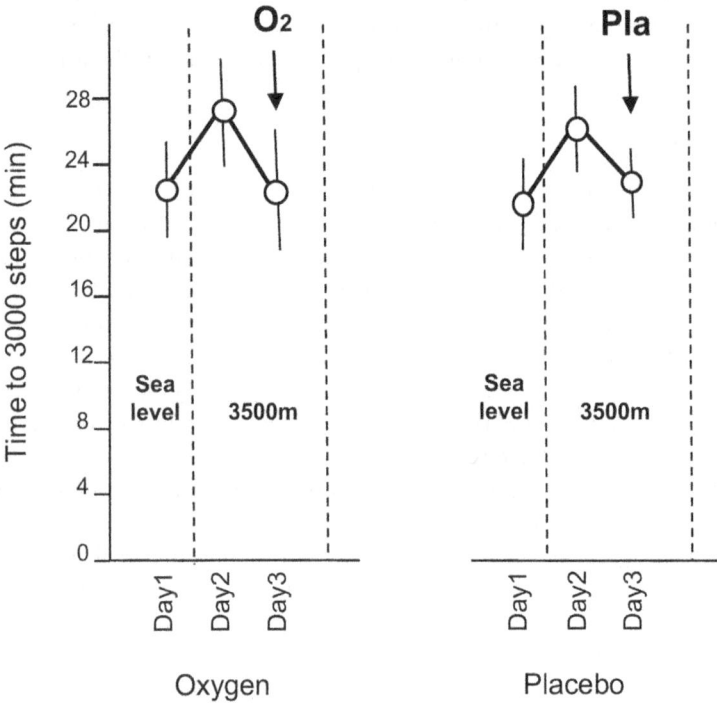

FIGURE 8.4 Here performance is measured as the time needed to complete 3000 steps on a stepper. It can be seen that in the subjects of the oxygen group time increases (performance worsens) from sea level to an altitude of 3500 m, but oxygen administration restores sea level performance. In the placebo group, a placebo produced the same effects as oxygen.

"first-time" placebo administration was sufficient to reduce perceived fatigue and increase performance. Therefore, the increase in SO2 after oxygen delivery was not completely responsible for the decrease in time to complete 3000 steps, as performance improved also with a placebo and without any SO2 increase.

In a simulation of high-altitude hypoxia in the lab at the sea level (Torres-Peralta et al., 2016), volunteers exercised in severe acute hypoxia (oxygen = 73mmHg). Upon exhaustion, subjects were asked to continue exercising while the breathing gas mixture was swiftly changed to a placebo (oxygen = 73 mmHg) or to 82, 92, 99, and 142 mmHg, and the exercise continued until a new exhaustion. At the second exhaustion, the breathing gas was changed to room air (normoxia) and the exercise continued until the final exhaustion. The switch to a placebo or higher oxygen pressures allowed for the continuation of exercise in all instances. The fact that at exhaustion in severe hypoxia the exercise was continued with the placebo-gas mixture demonstrates that a central and psychological mechanism is of crucial importance for performance.

The nocebo effect

No specific study of the nocebo effect at high altitude has been done in relation to oxygenation and ventilation. Inducing nocebo effects in these extreme and dangerous conditions would be unethical. However, within this context it is worth mentioning the effects of nocebo and negative expectations of some physiological and biochemical parameters that have been measured at high altitude. For example, it has been shown that the cyclooxygenase-prostaglandins (COX-PG) pathway can be modulated by nocebos (Benedetti et al., 2014). In fact, negative expectations about headache pain, the crucial element of the nocebo effect, leads to the enhancement of the COX-PG pathway which, in turn, induces pain worsening. It is interesting to note that PGE2 and headache are particularly sensitive to nocebo, which suggests that nocebos may affect cerebral vasodilation, as already discussed for placebos (see above). Thus, this could be considered as indirect evidence that nocebos, namely, negative expectations, may influence cerebral perfusion.

Conclusions and future challenges

Physiological functions, such as ventilation and heart rate, and other parameters, such as headache and performance, show placebo effects when oxygen is as low as 50% compared to sea level. The reduction of all these functions by oxygen is accompanied by an increase of SO2. By contrast, no SO2 increase is induced by placebo, yet this can influence some parameters in different ways. Fatigue and overall performance are very sensitive to placebo alone; that is, a placebo given for the first time along with verbal suggestions of reduced fatigue and improved performance. Instead, verbal suggestions alone have no effect on all the other parameters. However, if placebo is given after prior oxygen conditioning, a response also occurs for ventilation, blood pH, heart activity, PGE2, and post-exercise headache, thus indicating that learning plays a crucial role in these responses. The fact that these placebo effects take place without any change in SO2 suggests that psychobiological mechanisms are sometimes, and, in some circumstances, more important than or as important as the oxygen content of the body. The future challenge is threefold. First, we need to understand how these physiological placebo effects occur and how they can bypass the oxygen shortage in the body. Second, we need to identify the limits of these placebo effects, for oxygen reductions beyond 50%. Third, we need to analyse other physiological and biochemical parameters in order to understand which body functions are affected by placebos.

References

Bärtsch, P., Waber, U., Baumgartner, R., Maggiorini, M., & Oelz, O. (1990). Comparison of carbon-dioxide-enriched, oxygen-enriched, and normal air in treatment of acute mountain sickness. *The Lancet, 336*(8718), 772–775.

Benedetti, F. (2020). *Placebo effects.* Oxford University Press.

Benedetti, F., Amanzio, M., Rosato, R., & Blanchard, C. (2011). Nonopioid placebo analgesia is mediated by CB1 cannabinoid receptors. *Nature Medicine, 17*(10), 1228–1230.

Benedetti, F., Barbiani, D., & Camerone, E. (2018). Critical life functions: Can placebo replace oxygen? *International Review of Neurobiology, 138*, 201–218.

Benedetti, F., & Dogue, S. (2015). Different placebos, different mechanisms, different outcomes: Lessons for clinical trials. *PloS One, 10*(11), e0140967.

Benedetti, F., Durando, J., Giudetti, L., Pampallona, A., & Vighetti, S. (2015). High-altitude headache: The effects of real vs sham oxygen administration. *Pain, 156*(11), 2326–2336.

Benedetti, F., Durando, J., & Vighetti, S. (2014). Nocebo and placebo modulation of hypobaric hypoxia headache involves the cyclooxygenase-prostaglandins pathway. *Pain®, 155*(5), 921–928.

Burtscher, M., Likar, R., Nachbauer, W., & Philadelphy, M. (1998). Aspirin for prophylaxis against headache at high altitudes: Randomised, double blind, placebo controlled trial. *BMJ, 316*(7137), 1057.

Busse, R., Förstermann, U., Matsuda, H., & Pohl, U. (1984). The role of prostaglandins in the endothelium-mediated vasodilatory response to hypoxia. *Pflügers Archiv, 401*(1), 77–83.

de la Fuente-Fernández, R., Schulzer, M., & Stoessl, A. J. (2002). The placebo effect in neurological disorders. *The Lancet Neurology, 1*(2), 85–91.

De La Fuente-Fernandez, R., & Stoessl, A. J. (2002). The placebo effect in Parkinson's disease. *Trends in Neurosciences, 25*(6), 302–306.

Fredricks, K., Liu, Y., Rusch, N. J., & Lombard, J. H. (1994). Role of endothelium and arterial K+ channels in mediating hypoxic dilation of middle cerebral arteries. *American Journal of Physiology-Heart and Circulatory Physiology, 267*(2), H580–H586.

Hurst, P., Schiphof-Godart, L., Raglin, J., Coleman, D., Lane, A., Foad, A., & Beedie, C. (2019). Placebo effects on Sports Performance: A Systematic Review. *European Journal of Sport Science*. https://doi.org/10.1080/17461391.2019.1655098

Imray, C., Wright, A., Subudhi, A., & Roach, R. (2010). Acute mountain sickness: Pathophysiology, prevention, and treatment. *Progress in Cardiovascular Diseases*, 52(6), 467–484.

International Society for Mountain Medicine. (2017). http://www.ismm.org/index.php/normal-acclimatization.html

Kawabata, A., 2011. Prostaglandin E2 and pain—an update. *Biological and Pharmaceutical Bulletin*, 34(8), 1170–1173.

Krogh, A., & Lindhard, J. (1913). The regulation of respiration and circulation during the initial stages of muscular work. *The Journal of Physiology*, 47(1–2), 112.

Leaf, D. E., & Goldfarb, D. S. (2007). Mechanisms of action of acetazolamide in the prophylaxis and treatment of acute mountain sickness. *Journal of Applied Physiology*, 102, 1313–1322.

Messina, E., Sun, D., Koller, A., Wolin, M., & Kaley, G. (1992). Role of endothelium-derived prostaglandins in hypoxia-elicited arteriolar dilation in rat skeletal muscle. *Circulation Research*, 71(4), 790–796.

Noakes, T. D., St Clair Gibson, A., & Lambert, E. V. (2005). From catastrophe to complexity: A novel model of integrative central neural regulation of effort and fatigue during exercise in humans: Summary and conclusions. *British Journal of Sports Medicine*, 39(2), 120–124.

Petrovic, P., Kalso, E., Petersson, K. M., & Ingvar, M. (2002). Placebo and opioid analgesia--imaging a shared neuronal network. *Science*, 295(5560), 1737–1740.

Piedimonte, A., Benedetti, F., & Carlino, E. (2015). Placebo-induced decrease in fatigue: Evidence for a central action on the preparatory phase of movement. *European Journal of Neuroscience*, 41(4), 492–497.

Ray, C. J., Abbas, M. R., Coney, A. M., & Marshall, J. M. (2002). Interactions of adenosine, prostaglandins and nitric oxide in hypoxia-induced vasodilatation: In vivo and in vitro studies. *The Journal of Physiology*, 544(1), 195–209.

Richalet, J.-P., Hornych, A., Rathat, C., Aumont, J., Larmignat, P., & Remy, P. (1991). Plasma prostaglandins, leukotrienes and thromboxane in acute high altitude hypoxia. *Respiration Physiology*, 85(2), 205–215.

Schmidt, R., & Thews, G. (1989). *Human physiology*. Springer.

St Clair Gibson, A., Baden, D. A., Lambert, M. I., Lambert, E. V., Harley, Y. X., Hampson, D., Russell, V. A., & Noakes, T. D. (2003). The conscious perception of the sensation of fatigue. *Sports Medicine*, 33, 167–176.

St Clair Gibson, A., Lambert, E. V., Rauch, L. H., Tucker, R., Baden, D. A., Foster, C., & Noakes, T. D. (2006). The role of information processing between the brain and peripheral physiological systems in pacing and perception of effort. *Sports Medicine*, 36, 705–722.

Sutton, J., Coates, G., Houston, C., & Oelz, O. (1992). The Lake Louise consensus on the definition and quantification of altitude illness. In J. Coates, G. Sutton, & C. Houston (Eds.), *Hypoxia and mountain medicine* (pp. 327–330). Queen City Printers.

Torres-Peralta, R., Losa-Reyna, J., Morales-Alamo, D., González-Izal, M., Pérez-Suárez, I., Ponce-González, J. G., Izquierdo, M., & Calbet, J. A. (2016). Increased PIO2 at exhaustion in hypoxia enhances muscle activation and swiftly relieves fatigue: A placebo or a PIO2 dependent effect? *Frontiers in Physiology*, 7, 333.

West, J. B. (2005). The physiologic basis of high-altitude diseases. *Annals of Internal Medicine, 142*(7), 592.

Wilson, M. H., Newman, S., & Imray, C. H. (2009). The cerebral effects of ascent to high altitudes. *The Lancet Neurology, 8*(2), 175–191.

Wyss-Dunant, E. (1953). Acclimatisation. In M. Kurz (Ed.), *The mountain world.* Harper & Brothers.

9

CAN WE REMOVE PLACEBO EFFECTS FROM EXERCISE INTERVENTIONS?

Methodological considerations for understanding the psychological benefits of exercise

Jacob B. Lindheimer

Introduction

Exercise and physical activity are proposed to enhance psychological factors relating to quality of life (Martin et al., 2009), mental health (Cooney et al., 2013), and mental performance, what has often been termed the 'feelgood factor' of exercise. Meta-analytic reviews of randomised controlled trials of exercise indicate small to moderate improvements in self-reported psychological variables such as anxiety, depression, fatigue, and pain (Cooney et al., 2013; Herring et al., 2010; Herring et al., 2012; Puetz et al., 2006; Searle et al., 2015), and small effects on several components of cognitive performance (Smith et al., 2010). These findings appear to mirror research findings relating to the effects of exercise in physical health variables such as cardiorespiratory fitness, metabolic function, and physical function.

The importance of exercise has long been recognised in physical health, with physical inactivity identified as a leading cause of disease and death worldwide (Katzmarzyk et al., 2022). Research findings in relation to exercise and psychological outcomes are however equally important; not only are the psychological effects of exercise a core, if not critical factor in the adoption and maintenance of exercise for physical health, but the significant and often-meaningful antidepressant and anxiolytic effects reported in exercise studies are the basis on which many governments, health agencies, and medical institutions propose exercise as either an adjunct or standalone treatment for poor mental health and for mental illness. Increasingly, it is becoming clear that, as is the case in physical health, physical inactivity is also a factor in mental illness (Kandola & Osborn, 2022).

DOI: 10.4324/9781003229001-9

Mechanisms proposed to explain the psychological effects of exercise vary from social-cognitive factors such as distraction, physiological processes such as changes in neurotransmitter action, and anatomical effects such as neurogenesis (a change in the anatomical status and function of brain regions, for example the hippocampus involved in memory and emotion). Many studies attest to these effects (Ekkekakis et al., 2013).

It has also often been proposed that, as is the case with many health interventions elsewhere (Peerdeman et al., 2016), expectation plays a mechanistic role in the effects of exercise on psychological variables. That is, placebo effects might be associated with the benefits of exercise. This makes intuitive sense, and when we consider the relatively large number of studies that have investigated the placebo effect in sports performance (Hurst et al., 2020), it is reasonable to anticipate that an equivalent number of studies might have done likewise in relation to exercise. But as we'll see, studying the placebo effect of exercise is no simple thing, from either a conceptual or methodological perspective.

In this chapter, while the existing research is described, issues relating to the problematic research methodology associated with the study of placebo effects in exercise are used as a vehicle to help the reader better understand the role of expectation in exercise (and it is hoped to encourage higher quality research in the future). For practitioners and exercisers alike, it is hoped that a greater understanding of placebo effects in exercise will lead to improved understanding of the psychology of exercise more generally and thereby to enhanced benefits, psychological and physical, in very real terms.

Estimating the placebo effects of exercise

Until 2015 research into exercise and placebo effects had been sporadic, perhaps reflecting the status in placebo effect research in sports performance 10 years earlier. Lindheimer et al. (2015) reviewed the literature, specifically to quantify the mean effect size of placebo effects across randomised controlled trials of exercise compared to the overall observed effect of exercise itself (in short, to establish what percentage of the effect of exercise is a placebo). To be included in the meta-analysis, studies were required to meet two criteria: (i) used a design that randomly assigned participants to exercise training, placebo, *and* control conditions; and (ii) reported an assessment of a subjective (i.e., anxiety, depression, energy, fatigue) or an objective (i.e., cognitive) psychological outcome. Data from nine studies involving 661 participants were included, and authors reported a mean effect size for the placebo effect of exercise at 0.20 (95% CI, –0.02, 0.41) against an overall effect size of exercise at 0.37 (95% CI, 0.11, 0.63). The authors concluded that the placebo effect of exercise interventions, reported in well-designed research trials, was *approximately half of the observed psychological benefits of exercise training,* and that

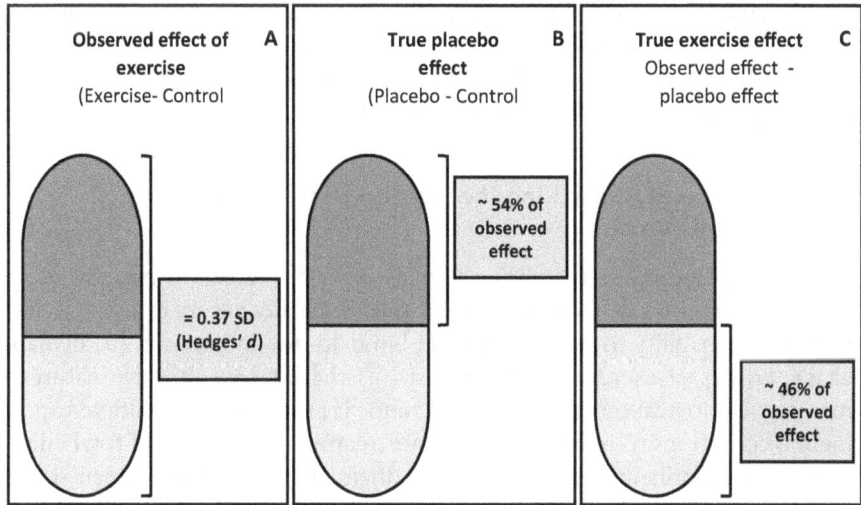

FIGURE 9.1　Distinguishing the true effect of exercise on psychological responses from non-specific effects requires the inclusion of a placebo and no-treatment control group. Panel A shows what is typically measured in exercise studies, the observed effect of exercise, which is estimated by comparing the change in the exercise group to the control group. Panel B shows the true placebo effect, which is estimated by comparing the change in the placebo group to the control group. Panel C shows that the true effect of exercise can be estimated by subtracting the true placebo effect from the observed effect of exercise. In a meta-analysis of randomised controlled studies that included an exercise, placebo, and control group, approximately half of the observed effect of exercise on psychological outcomes was attributed to placebo effects (Lindheimer et al., 2015).

there is an urgent need for creative research specifically aimed at better understanding the role of the placebo effect in the mental health consequences of exercise training (Figure 9.1).

The conclusion that ~50% of the effects of exercise on psychological outcomes is a placebo effect is, at first sight, a provocative suggestion, not only for advocates of and participants in exercise, but also for exercise and sports medicine professionals, health agencies, and medical institutions who promote exercise for its therapeutic effects. But to contextualise the finding, previous research in mental health suggests that the placebo effect of antidepressants is higher still at around 75% (Kirsch & Sapirstein, 1999), so while the idea of 50% of the effects of exercise being a placebo might appear initially challenging, it is not without precedent. In fact, when this effect is interrogated objectively, it speaks more to the complexity of human psychological function and to the myriad systems involved in promoting health and wellbeing than it does any deficit in the effects of exercise. But it also suggests that the psychological effects of exercise might be enhanced through the modification of people's expectations of exercise, and that is a potentially useful idea for all involved in exercise promotion, especially in mental health.

The challenges of researching the placebo effect of exercise on psychological outcomes

Unlike the placebo effects of drugs such as antidepressants, the placebo effects of exercise are not easy to quantify. Four specific challenges are evident, including: (i) the inability to perform double-blind studies in exercise; (ii) demand characteristics of exercise interventions; (iii) the largely subjective nature of many psychological outcome measures; and (iv) the need for multiple experimental conditions to reliably compare no-treatment, placebo and total effects of exercise (Lindheimer et al., 2015; Lindheimer et al., 2020; Ojanen, 1994; Szabo, 2013).

Challenge 1: The inability to perform double-blind studies

Unlike many, if not most health interventions such as drugs, surgery, and psychotherapy, it is problematic to engineer an equivalent comparison treatment for exercise that also controls for placebo effects. That is, unlike a drug which can be replaced with an inert substance, surgery that can be replaced with a procedure that does not involve replacement or repair, or a counselling session that can be replaced with a sham script, it is challenging to the point of being impossible, to deliver a legitimate sham exercise intervention. This is largely due to someone knowing that they are exercising. Given this, the proposal that exercise exerts some, most, or even the entirety of its effect on psychological functions via placebo effects is therefore not easy to support, or indeed challenge, empirically.

Challenge 2: Demand characteristics

It is probably not all that surprising to learn that the majority of people who volunteer to participate in a study of exercise and psychological variables expect the exercise to have an effect. Even if this expectation isn't the result of any explicit knowledge or information, most participants will probably accept that the scientists are studying the phenomena for a reason, and that sets up an expectation that something will change. Such factors are called ***demand characteristics***, the totality of cues that can lead a participant to guess the experimental hypothesis of the study (Orne, 1962). A significant source of these cues can arise from study materials (e.g., advertisements, informed consent documents).

For instance, Foroughi and colleagues reported that following one hour of practicing cognitive tasks, performance on fluid intelligence tests was better among participants who enrolled in the study after viewing an overt advertisement for a "Brain Training and Cognitive Enhancement Study" compared to participants who responded to a generic advertisement with no information about brain training or cognitive enhancement (Foroughi et al., 2016). Although the authors did not collect explicit information that would allow them to test for between-group differences in expectations, their study provided a clear example of how information that overtly communicates the study purpose can affect a given participant's behaviour. This issue is rarely considered in exercise research, with one exception. One study reported an attempt to control for this particular demand characteristic by using deceptive information in the study advertisement and informed consent materials (Lindheimer et al., 2017). Interestingly, the authors did not report a significant effect of exercise on the study outcomes (e.g., feelings of energy, state anxiety, and working memory), thus highlighting the importance of paying close attention to the messages that study advertisements and informed consent documents may communicate to participants.

Demand characteristics can also stem from interactions between test administrators and study participants. For instance, consider a clinical trial that examines the effect of exercise training on cognitive performance compared to a no-treatment control condition. A test administrator may inadvertently bias a participant who they know is in the exercise group to try harder on the cognitive task than those assigned to the control group because of their own inherent bias that exercise will improve cognition. To prevent this situation from occurring, an investigator can try implementing a single blinding procedure by ensuring that study personnel who are involved in exercise training are not also involved in test administration. Indeed, the role of demand characteristics in psychological responses to exercise has long been recognised (Morgan, 1997) and relatively feasible strategies such as using neutral language in study materials and blinding test administrators can be used to minimise their effects. As an alternative, researchers can ask participants to rate on a Likert-type scale how much they expect the exercise to improve the outcome in question and include this as a covariate in the analysis. For example, researchers could ask participants "How much do you agree with the following statement: 'the exercise will improve my anxiety'?" on a scale of 1 (strongly disagree) to 5 (strongly agree). Collectively, while these steps may increase the methodological rigor of exercise research, they are not always practical to implement and unlikely to completely prevent study-specific expectations from developing. Thus, even the most well-designed studies should consider including measures of expectations to better understand their potential influence on the results.

Challenge 3: The subjective nature of psychological outcome variables

Many of the effects of exercise can be seen as objectively measurable and operating in a dose–response manner, for example changes in energy expenditure resulting from exercise can not only be directly measured but can be observed in concomitant changes in body composition. Some ostensibly physiological changes such as a reduction in blood pressure have a subjective component, meaning that subjective status might modify them (for example, anxiety can increase blood pressure), while many, if not most purported psychological effects can only be accessed via self-report. These include mental health variables such as anxiety and depression, affective variables such as mood and emotion, perceptual variables such as rating of perceived exertion (RPE), muscle pain, pain intensity, and symptom severity, and self-referenced constructs such as body image and self-esteem. Even cognitive factors such as attention and memory are not entirely objective measures. Therefore, it must be recognised that any inferences made from psychometric measures are susceptible to subjective bias, and may not be a result of the intervention or placebo effects.

Challenge 4: The need for multiple experimental conditions

The importance of designing exercise-based studies to account for placebo effects was recognised over three decades ago (McCann & Holmes, 1984); however, progress toward advancing the current standard of knowledge about placebo effects and their respective mechanisms in psychological responses to exercise has been relatively slow compared to other scientific fields. Part of the problem is that it is difficult to reliably estimate the magnitude of placebo effects in randomised controlled trials when both a placebo *and* control comparison group are not included (Ernst & Resch, 1995). The introduction of the terms *placebo effects* and *placebo responses* has helped clarify why this is the case (Evers et al., 2018; see also Raglin's chapter in this book). An early misconception was that placebo effects could be studied by measuring change from baseline in the placebo group (i.e., perceived placebo effect; Beecher, 1955). However, this approach fails to consider that changes in a placebo group can result from non-specific effects such as natural history of disease, regression towards the mean, and unidentified parallel interventions (Ernst & Resch, 1995; Kienle & Kiene, 1997). Presumably, these same effects have an equal likelihood of occurring in a wait-list or no-treatment control group; therefore, placebo responses are measured by comparing the change in the placebo group to that of the control group and related to changes in outcome measures after administration of a placebo (i.e., differences in symptoms before and after treatment). Whereas, *placebo effect*s are changes attributable to placebo mechanisms, including the neurobiological and psychological mechanisms following the administration of a placebo.

Given the above, in the exercise setting, the terms placebo responses and placebo effects are synonymous with *observed effect of exercise* and *true effect of exercise* (Ojanen, 1994). That is, in a group that has been assigned to receive the exercise treatment, the observed effect of exercise is the psychological response resulting from both true effects of exercise and placebo effects whereas the true effect of exercise is the psychological response that can be solely attributed to the exercise *per se*. Consequently, to obtain the most precise estimation of the effect of exercise on psychological responses in a clinical trial or randomised controlled study design, we use the principles outlined by Ernst & Resch (1995) and Ojanen (1994) to offer the following guidelines:

- Determining the true effect of exercise/true treatment effect requires separation of the placebo effect from the observed effect of exercise/perceived treatment effect.
- In order to distinguish the placebo effect from the placebo response, a no-treatment or wait-list control group is needed to rule out non-specific effects that may explain changes in the outcome measure over time.
- Obtaining the most precise estimation of the true effect of exercise/true treatment effect in a clinical trial or randomised controlled study design requires that participants be allocated to at least three groups – treatment, placebo, and control.

Research designs to elucidate mechanisms of placebo effects in exercise

Most of the data concerning placebo and placebo-related effects in psychological responses to exercise have been generated from the few three-arm intervention studies that have included an exercise, placebo, and control condition, or from two-arm studies that have compared outcome expectations between the exercise and control group. While germane to facilitating the broader understanding of placebo effects and placebo responses in exercise, these types of study designs are not well suited to elucidating psychological and neurobiological mechanisms.

An illuminating review by Benedetti and colleagues has distinguished the application and objectives of studying placebo effects in the clinical trial setting from the experimental-laboratory setting – "whereas the clinical trialist is interested in any improvement that may take place in a clinical trial, the neurobiologist is only interested in the psychosocial-psychobiological effects after the administration of a placebo" (Benedetti, Carlino, et al., 2011). Thus, while clinical trials are useful for understanding the magnitude of placebo effects and placebo responses, laboratory-based studies contribute information about the potential mechanisms underlying these effects. The next section of this chapter discusses several study designs with potential to advance the understanding of mechanisms of placebo effects and placebo responses in psychological outcomes of exercise.

Expectancy modification

A well-established model for studying expectations as a psychological mechanism of placebo effects is the *expectancy modification* design, which uses situational or behavioural cues to create or augment the belief that a certain outcome will occur (Kirsch, 1985). Expectancy modification is the most frequently adopted strategy for studying placebo mechanisms in exercise (Crum & Langer, 2007; Desharnais et al., 1993; Helfer et al., 2015; Kwan et al., 2017; Lindheimer et al., 2017; Mothes, Leukel, Jo, et al., 2017; Mothes, Leukel, Seelig, et al., 2017). In exercise studies, the expectancy modification procedure is typically used to induce placebo-related effects by experimentally augmenting the belief that exercise will result in a given psychological outcome. Following expectancy modification, psychological responses to exercise in participants in the experimental condition are compared to control condition participants whose expectations were not modified.

Various strategies such as verbal suggestion (Crum & Langer, 2007; Desharnais et al., 1993; Helfer et al., 2015; Lindheimer et al., 2017; McCann & Holmes, 1984), film clips (Mothes, Leukel, Jo, et al., 2017; Mothes, Leukel, Seelig, et al., 2017), and reading standardised scripts (Kwan et al., 2017) have been used to manipulate expectations. In some cases, these modifications have been further enhanced through additional psychosocial and environmental cues (Crum & Langer, 2007; Desharnais et al., 1993) or engagement of conscious mental processes by asking participants to recapitulate and record their expectations (Helfer et al., 2015; Kwan et al., 2017). It is not yet clear which types of modification procedures are most effective for influencing expectations about psychological outcomes of exercise. To help address this gap, studies can incorporate *manipulation checks* by measuring and comparing expectations between the experimental and control group to provide insight into why some studies are more successful with manipulating expectations (Desharnais et al., 1993) than others (Lindheimer et al., 2017).

The balanced placebo design

A special case of an expectancy modification study is the *balanced placebo design* (Rohsenow & Marlatt, 1981; Ross et al., 1962). By assigning participants to a drug or placebo condition and manipulating their expectations

TABLE 9.1 The balanced placebo design is a model for observing expectancy-related placebo effects that can be adapted to studying psychological responses to exercise if a valid exercise placebo is ever developed. Study participants are randomised to a treatment or inert/sham condition and half of the participants in each condition are subjected to an expectancy modification procedure that is designed to increase expectations for psychological improvements following the exposure to the treatment or inert/sham stimulus

Balanced placebo design		Type of stimulus	
		Sham/inert	Treatment
Expectancy manipulation	No information about psychological effects of stimulus provided	Inert stimulus (Control)	Active stimulus (Treatment effect)
	Receive information about psychological effects of stimulus	Inert stimulus + information (Placebo effect)	Active stimulus + information (Treatment effect + placebo effect)

about condition assignment, this design allows the investigator to differentiate between the treatment effect (i.e., participants who receive the treatment, but are told they received the placebo) and placebo effect (i.e., participants who receive the placebo, but are told they received the treatment) (Table 9.1).

The balanced placebo design was developed for researching expectancy effects in drug responses (Enck et al., 2011), but it has also been modified to the study of placebo effects in psychological responses to exercise. Using a recumbent motorised cycle to provide either a sham/inert or treatment stimulus, Lindheimer and colleagues assigned participants to a passive condition in which participants' legs were involuntarily moved for them (i.e., sham/inert) or an active condition in which participants cycled under their own volition (i.e., treatment; Lindheimer et al., 2017). Additionally, half of participants in each condition were exposed to an expectancy modification procedure to generate expectations that active or passive cycling would result in post-treatment improvements in mood and cognitive performance.

Conditioning

A powerful psychological mechanism of placebo effects that is untested in exercise studies is conditioning. Placebo conditioning has been studied in a variety of settings (Hadamitzky et al., 2018), and one directly relevant application to this review is conditioned placebo hypoalgesia (i.e., increased sensitivity to pain). Following an initial familiarisation period during which participants are introduced to a painful stimulus (unconditioned stimulus), placebo hypo-algesia can be conditioned by pairing the administration of a placebo (conditioned stimulus) with surreptitious reduction of the pain stimulus intensity. This is often repeated several times to ensure that the conditioned response to the placebo has taken effect (Colloca et al., 2010), and is followed by an experimental phase to examine the strength and duration of the placebo effect. In order to do so, the full-intensity painful stimulus is re-administered and perceptual ratings are compared between participants who received the conditioning procedure and a control group who did not. By repeatedly conducting the experimental phase over the course of several days, the investigator can also determine the time-course for the conditioned placebo response to be extinguished.

Conditioning represents a promising approach to studying placebo effects in exercise, particularly in the study of exercise-induced hypoalgesia, a phenomenon in which pain sensitivity is reduced during or following exercise (Koltyn, 2002). This area of inquiry is especially intriguing because exercise-induced hypoalgesia and placebo hypoalgesia appear to involve similar bio-chemical mechanisms such as the opioid and endocannabinoid systems (Benedetti, Amanzio, et al., 2011; Crombie et al., 2018). Yet, despite extensive interest among both exercise and placebo researchers in studying pain, no studies have been designed to explore placebo effects or placebo-related effects in exercise induced hypoalgesia.

Future directions

The understanding of the role of outcome expectations in psychological responses to exercise could be further improved by developing psychometrically validated instruments that assess specific expectations for positive and negative psychological changes. It would also be useful to determine the extent to which positive and negative expectations are moderated by factors such as preferred mode of exercise (e.g., running, cycling, swimming, weightlifting), self-reported physical activity behaviour, and cardio-respiratory fitness. These data would provide insight into the role that the stimulus characteristics of exercise play in the psychosocial factors that trigger placebo effects.

Until a valid exercise placebo is developed, it is not possible to investigate mechanisms of placebo effects in psychological outcomes of exercise. However, mechanisms of placebo-related effects can be investigated with expectancy-modification and conditioning studies. These designs can be used to explore potential biological mechanisms that are involved in amplifying the effect of exercise on psychological outcomes. Expectancy modification studies are encouraged to test for within-group changes over time or between-group differences in study-specific expectations as a manipulation check. Aside from the importance of verifying the success of the manipulation, this information would allow researchers to begin cataloguing which types of expectancy modi-fication procedures are most effective. Conditioning studies are a promising strategy for investigating mechanisms of placebo-related effects in certain psy-chological outcomes of exercise, especially pain. Further insight into whether it is possible to condition placebo responses to inert minimal exercise modali-ties such as passive cycling would provide preliminary evidence that exercise placebos can be used to study placebo effects in laboratory settings and pos-sibly even clinical trial settings.

Conclusions

Distinguishing the effect of exercise from placebo effects requires a placebo group. While efforts to develop a valid exercise placebo are underway, research-ers can capitalise on using established psychological mechanisms of placebo effects to better understand how psychosocial context influences psychological responses to exercise in clinical trials and laboratory settings. Measuring out-come expectations in clinical trials can help explain inter-individual variability in positive and negative outcomes of exercise and this information may help design more effective exercise interventions in the future. Expectancy-modification and conditioning designs can be used in laboratory studies to help elucidate the mechanisms that are involved in placebo-related effects. These endeavours would make a valuable contribution toward advancing the current standard of knowledge about placebo and placebo-related effects in psychological responses to exercise.

Acknowledgements

This work was supported in part by Career Development Award Number IK2 CX001679 from the United States (U.S.) Department of Veterans Affairs Clinical Sciences R&D (CSRD) Service. The contents do not represent the views of the Department of Veterans Affairs or the United States Government

References

Beecher, H. K. (1955). The powerful placebo. *Journal of the American Medical Association*, *159*(17), 1602–1606.

Benedetti, F., Amanzio, M., Rosato, R., & Blanchard, C. (2011). Nonopioid placebo analgesia is mediated by CB1 cannabinoid receptors. *Nature Medicine*, *17*(10), 1228–1230.

Benedetti, F., Carlino, E., & Pollo, A. (2011). How placebos change the patient's brain. *Neuropsychopharmacology*, *36*(1), 339–354.

Colloca, L., Petrovic, P., Wager, T. D., Ingvar, M., & Benedetti, F. (2010). How the number of learning trials affects placebo and nocebo responses. *Pain*®, *151*(2), 430–439.

Cooney, G. M., Dwan, K., Greig, C. A., Lawlor, D. A., Rimer, J., Waugh, F. R., McMurdo, M., & Mead, G. E. (2013). Exercise for depression. *Cochrane Database of Systematic Reviews*, 2013(9), CD004366. doi: 10.1002/14651858.CD004366. pub6.

Crombie, K. M., Brellenthin, A. G., Hillard, C. J., & Koltyn, K. F. (2018). Endocannabinoid and opioid system interactions in exercise-induced hypoalgesia. *Pain Medicine*, 19(1), 118–123.

Crum, A. J., & Langer, E. J. (2007). Mind-set matters: Exercise and the placebo effect. *Psychological Science*, 18(2), 165–171.

Desharnais, R., Jobin, J., Côté, C., Lévesque, L., & Godin, G. (1993). Aerobic exercise and the placebo effect: A controlled study. *Psychosomatic Medicine*, 55(2), 149–154.

Ekkekakis, P. E., Cook, D. B., Craft, L. L., Culos-Reed, S., Etnier, J. L., Hamer, M. E., Martin Ginis, K. A., Reed, J. E., Smits, J. A., & Ussher, M. E. (2013). *Routledge handbook of physical activity and mental health*. Routledge/Taylor & Francis Group.

Enck, P., Klosterhalfen, S., & Zipfel, S. (2011). Novel study designs to investigate the placebo response. *BMC Medical Research Methodology*, 11(1), 1–8.

Ernst, E., & Resch, K. L. (1995). Concept of true and perceived placebo effects. *BMJ*, 311(7004), 551–553.

Evers, A. W., Colloca, L., Blease, C., Annoni, M., Atlas, L. Y., Benedetti, F., Bingel, U., Büchel, C., Carvalho, C., & Colagiuri, B. (2018). Implications of placebo and nocebo effects for clinical practice: Expert consensus. *Psychotherapy and Psychosomatics*, 87(4), 204–210.

Foroughi, C. K., Monfort, S. S., Paczynski, M., McKnight, P. E., & Greenwood, P. (2016). Placebo effects in cognitive training. *Proceedings of the National Academy of Sciences*, 113(27), 7470–7474.

Hadamitzky, M., Sondermann, W., Benson, S., & Schedlowski, M. (2018). Placebo effects in the immune system. *International Review of Neurobiology*, 138, 39–59.

Helfer, S. G., Elhai, J. D., & Geers, A. L. (2015). Affect and exercise: Positive affective expectations can increase post-exercise mood and exercise intentions. *Annals of Behavioral Medicine*, 49(2), 269–279.

Herring, M. P., O'Connor, P. J., & Dishman, R. K. (2010). The effect of exercise training on anxiety symptoms among patients: A systematic review. *Archives of Internal Medicine*, 170(4), 321–331.

Herring, M. P., Puetz, T. W., O'Connor, P. J., & Dishman, R. K. (2012). Effect of exercise training on depressive symptoms among patients with a chronic illness: A systematic review and meta-analysis of randomized controlled trials. *Archives of Internal Medicine*, 172(2), 101–111.

Hurst, P., Schipof-Godart, L., Szabo, A., Raglin, J., Hettinga, F., Roelands, B., Lane, A., Foad, A., Coleman, D., & Beedie, C. (2020). The placebo and nocebo effect on sports performance: A systematic review. *European Journal of Sport Science*, 20(3), 279–292.

Kandola, A. A., & Osborn, D. P. (2022). Physical activity as an intervention in severe mental illness. *BJPsych Advances*, 28(2), 112–121.

Katzmarzyk, P. T., Friedenreich, C., Shiroma, E. J., & Lee, I.-M. (2022). Physical inactivity and non-communicable disease burden in low-income, middle-income and high-income countries. *British Journal of Sports Medicine*, 56(2), 101–106.

Kienle, G. S., & Kiene, H. (1997). The powerful placebo effect: Fact or fiction? *Journal of Clinical Epidemiology*, *50*(12), 1311–1318.

Kirsch, I. (1985). Response expectancy as a determinant of experience and behavior. *American Psychologist*, *40*(11), 1189.

Kirsch, I., & Sapirstein, G. (1999). Listening to Prozac but hearing placebo: A meta-analysis of antidepressant medications.

Koltyn, K. F. (2002). Exercise-induced hypoalgesia and intensity of exercise. *Sports Medicine*, *32*, 477–487.

Kwan, B. M., Stevens, C. J., & Bryan, A. D. (2017). What to expect when you're exercising: An experimental test of the anticipated affect–exercise relationship. *Health Psychology*, *36*(4), 309.

Lindheimer, J. B., O'Connor, P. J., McCully, K. K., & Dishman, R. K. (2017). The effect of light-intensity cycling on mood and working memory in response to a randomized, placebo-controlled design. *Psychosomatic Medicine*, *79*(2), 243–253.

Lindheimer, J. B., O'Connor, P. J., & Dishman, R. K. (2015). Quantifying the placebo effect in psychological outcomes of exercise training: A meta-analysis of randomized trials. *Sports Medicine*, *45*, 693–711.

Lindheimer, J. B., Szabo, A., Raglin, J. S., & Beedie, C. (2020). Advancing the understanding of placebo effects in psychological outcomes of exercise: Lessons learned and future directions. *European Journal of Sport Science*, *20*(3), 326–337.

Martin, C. K., Church, T. S., Thompson, A. M., Earnest, C. P., & Blair, S. N. (2009). Exercise dose and quality of life: A randomized controlled trial. *Archives of Internal Medicine*, *169*(3), 269–278.

McCann, I. L., & Holmes, D. S. (1984). Influence of aerobic exercise on depression. *Journal of Personality and Social Psychology*, *46*(5), 1142.

Morgan, W. P. (1997). *Physical activity and mental health*. Taylor & Francis.

Mothes, H., Leukel, C., Jo, H.-G., Seelig, H., Schmidt, S., & Fuchs, R. (2017). Expectations affect psychological and neurophysiological benefits even after a single bout of exercise. *Journal of Behavioral Medicine*, *40*, 293–306.

Mothes, H., Leukel, C., Seelig, H., & Fuchs, R. (2017). Do placebo expectations influence perceived exertion during physical exercise? *PLoS One*, *12*(6), e0180434.

Ojanen, M. (1994). Can the true effects of exercise on psychological variables be separated from placebo effects? *International Journal of Sport Psychology*, *25*(1), 63–80.

Orne, M. T. (1962). On the social psychology of the psychological experiment: With particular reference to demand characteristics and their implications. *American Psychologist*, *17*(11), 776.

Peerdeman, K. J., van Laarhoven, A. I., Keij, S. M., Vase, L., Rovers, M. M., Peters, M. L., & Evers, A. W. (2016). Relieving patients' pain with expectation interventions: A meta-analysis. *Pain*, *157*(6), 1179–1191.

Puetz, T. W., O'Connor, P. J., & Dishman, R. K. (2006). Effects of chronic exercise on feelings of energy and fatigue: A quantitative synthesis. *Psychological Bulletin*, *132*(6), 866.

Rohsenow, D. J., & Marlatt, G. A. (1981). The balanced placebo design: Methodological considerations. *Addictive Behaviors*, *6*(2), 107–122.

Ross, S., Krugman, A. D., Lyerly, S. B., Clyde, J. D. (1962). Drugs and placebos: A model design. *Psychological Reports*, *10*(2), 383–392.

Searle, A., Spink, M., Ho, A., & Chuter, V. (2015). Exercise interventions for the treatment of chronic low back pain: A systematic review and meta-analysis of randomised controlled trials. *Clinical Rehabilitation, 29*(12), 1155–1167.

Smith, P. J., Blumenthal, J. A., Hoffman, B. M., Cooper, H., Strauman, T. A., Welsh-Bohmer, K., Browndyke, J. N., & Sherwood, A. (2010). Aerobic exercise and neurocognitive performance: A meta-analytic review of randomized controlled trials. *Psychosomatic Medicine, 72*(3), 239.

Szabo, A. (2013). Acute psychological benefits of exercise: Reconsideration of the placebo effect. *Journal of Mental Health, 22*(5), 449–455.

10

DO PLACEBO EFFECTS IMPROVE MY SKILL?

The influence of placebo effects on motor control and learning

Mirta Fiorio and Diletta Barbiani

Introduction

Motor performance is a multifaceted concept encompassing various dimensions, such as force production, precision control, movement speed, motor skill learning, resistance to fatigue, and motor adaptation. These motor skills are critical to human functioning because they impact an individual's ability to move independently and develop adaptive behaviors. Beyond everyday life, the refinement of motor skills is crucial in contexts in which they serve as indexes of "success", such as sports performance and pathological conditions. Indeed, the role of placebos in different motor domains has often been inferred from research in these fields, where placebos have been shown to be effective in enhancing athletic performance (Hurst et al., 2020) and improving motor symptoms in patient populations (Lidstone et al., 2010). When taking into account specific motor functions, most of these studies have adopted a "bottom-up" approach, whereby placebos disguised as effective treatments were targeted to treat or improve a condition "as a whole", and where effects on the motor domains specific for the condition in question were inferred accordingly. Contrarily, less appreciation has been devoted to "top-down" approaches, in which specific motor functions and/or skills are pinpointed *a priori* to be investigated in their own right under controlled laboratory conditions. For example, an in-depth understanding of how placebos may impact specific motor districts (e.g. upper limbs vs lower limbs) and their related functions is still lacking thorough investigation. As such, and to unpick the basic mechanisms of the placebo effect in specific domains and to broaden its potential applications and implications, evidence from controlled laboratory experiments during the execution of motor tasks is warranted.

DOI: 10.4324/9781003229001-10

The placebo effect on fine-tuned motor control of the hand and the upper limb

The majority of placebo effect studies in the motor domain have concerned whole-body performance, as in the field of sports. However, recent findings also point to the role of placebos for more fine and localised movements, such as those performed with either a single or a restricted muscle group. Falling under this domain are, for example, movements characterised by an abduction or flexion of the finger and upper limb. Narrowing the investigation to specific muscle districts not only allows an understanding of the neurophysiological processes, but also allows a more targeted translation of these findings in clinical and sports contexts.

The placebo effect on force control

In both everyday life and sports activities, we perform different types of movements ranging from fine movements of the hands or upper limb to more complex movements of the lower limbs and the entire body. As a result, a fine-tuning of both the generation and the relaxation of forces must be accurately performed such that one can move their body as intended. Importantly, especially during unfamiliar movements, relaxing the force in an appropriate manner could often require more effort than generating it. Thus, controlling force generation and relaxation accuracy is considered to be a basic and essential requirement (Kato et al., 2014; Spraker et al., 2009).

The role of placebos on force generation and control for movements performed with the upper limb has only recently started to gain appreciation. In particular, placebo procedures targeted to modulate force during upper-limb movements are proving effective even in healthy non-athletes individuals, as shown with different motor tasks, such as finger and arm movements (Bottoms et al., 2014; Fiorio et al., 2014; Fitts, 1954; Piedimonte et al., 2015; Rossettini et al., 2018).

Quite recently, Rossettini et al. (2018) investigated whether a placebo procedure applied at the level of the index finger would increase force when pressing against a piston, and whether this effect could be modulated by manipulating the focus of attention toward (i.e., internal focus) or away from (external focus) the movements of the finger. Healthy volunteers of the two placebo groups (i.e., one group with internal focus, the other with external focus) were asked to perform abduction movements with their index finger as strongly as possible after receiving an inert treatment (low-frequency transcutaneous electrical nerve stimulation [TENS]) over the hand muscle involved in the task (i.e., the first dorsal interosseous), along with positive suggestions that it would enhance force. Importantly, both placebo groups were visually conditioned through a surreptitious amplification of visual feedback signaling their "improved" level of force. Remarkably, only the placebo group in which attention was directed inwardly (toward the movement of the fingers) showed higher levels of force, whilst a decrease in force was observed for the group in which attention was directed outwardly (i.e., towards the movements of the piston). Moreover, electromyographical data showed that the former placebo group increased the muscle recruitment units without changing the neuronal firing rates, possibly indicating a persistence of force levels without muscle fatigue. Taken together, these findings suggest that force production at the level of a specific muscle district (first dorsal interosseus, FDI) may be influenced by a placebo procedure, even more so when the focus of attention is directed internally (Rossettini et al., 2018). These findings overwrite the ones of a previous study employing a similar procedure, without any attention manipulation but with the use of transcranial magnetic stimulation (TMS; Fiorio et al., 2014). Herein, the exposure to placebo suggestions combined with a conditioning paradigm with visual feedback improved force production at the level of the index finger, with changes being substantiated by an increased amplitude of the motor evoked potentials and a decreased duration of the cortical silent period. Crucially, these findings hint at a top-down, cognitive enhancement of corticospinal excitability as a neural marker of placebo modulation of motor performance.

Evidence that the placebo effect on force can be mediated at a central level comes from another study orientated on two other crucial components of motor performance, namely, the preparatory phase of movement and fatigue perception (Piedimonte et al., 2015). The aim of this study was to investigate whether a placebo disguised as endurance-increasing caffeine would induce changes in the readiness potential of the preparatory phase of movement during repeated flexions of the index finger compared to a no-treatment control. Results showed that the placebo group reported a decrease in perceived fatigue and no increase in readiness potential amplitude whereas the control group reported a concomitant increase in the amplitude of the readiness potential. This placebo-induced modulation of the readiness potential underscores that verbal suggestions may impact the preparatory phase of movement by acting at a central level, and that this mechanism could play an important part in the generation of fatigue, even for movements that engage small muscle districts.

In the context of upper-limb movements, two studies have investigated the effect of placebo administration on pain and fatigue of the arm and forearm. In a simulation of a sport competition, Benedetti et al. (2007) tested whether a preconditioning procedure with morphine in the pre-competition training phase would decrease pain tolerance and increase time to exhaustion during the squeeze and release of a hand-spring exerciser while applying the tourniquet technique to induce ischemic pain. Remarkably, a placebo (i.e., saline solution) injected on the day of the competition produced substantial increases in pain tolerance and physical performance (time to exhaustion of hand-spring movements) only in the group who underwent the morphine preconditioning training, underscoring how smaller placebo effects are achieved when a placebo is given for the first time as compared to when it is administered after a pharmacological preconditioning procedure.

Finally, one study investigated placebo and nocebo effects of an inert sugar-free drink depicted as being either 'performance-enhancing' (placebo) or 'fatigue-inducing' (nocebo) on peak minute power during incremental arm crank ergometry in three separate sessions spaced out by one week (Bottoms et al., 2014). Thirty minutes prior to the motor task, participants were asked to drink the beverages along with performance-enhancing (placebo) or performance-deteriorating (nocebo) suggestions. Results highlighted a significant increase in peak minute power during the arm crank ergometry task when participants ingested both placebo drinks as compared to water (control). However, a significant decrease in local ratings of perceived exertion were observed only in the group receiving positive suggestions and in neither of the nocebo and control groups. As such, the increase in performance in participants of the placebo group was higher and went hand in hand with a concomitant decrease in arm discomfort. These findings indicate that a placebo may influence sports performance, even for the smaller muscle mass of the arms, for which less pronounced effects would be expected as opposed to lower body exercises.

The placebo effect on goal-directed movements

Many daily activities, like picking up a cup of coffee or reaching for a bottle of water, require an optimal balance between movement precision and speed. The speed–accuracy trade-off for goal-directed actions has been described by Fitts (1954), who demonstrated that the time needed to execute a movement with the upper limb from a starting point to a final one depends on the distance and the size of the target to be reached. When the target is far away and small, the movement time is longer, whereas when the target is near and big, the movement time is shorter. Interestingly, a recent study (Fiorio et al., 2022) demonstrated that a placebo procedure (i.e., inert electrical device) disguised as an effective means for optimising movement precision can reduce forearm movement time toward a target than a control condition in which no precision-enhancing effects were emphasised. Remarkably, this effect was doubled after a second application of the placebo treatment, indicating a dose-dependent placebo response, a finding that is similar to that observed with previous studies on different tasks (Seidler et al., 2004). Moreover, perception of mental and physical fatigability was lower in the placebo compared to the control condition, pointing to placebo effects on both behavioral and subjective components of performance.

These findings may well be explained through the interplay between feedback and feedforward processes of motor control. Optimal movement control requires a combination of both inherently slow feedback process, in which sensory information is used to update ongoing movements, and more rapid feedforward processes, in which a pre-existing internal model of the movement allows to swiftly estimate the future sensory state of the moving limb (Desmurget & Grafton, 2000). In Fitts' task, these processes may alternate depending on the index of difficulty: when the task is difficult (i.e., the target is far and small), slow feedback processes prevail, while when the task is easy (i.e., the target is near and big), rapid feedforward processes can occur (Seidler et al., 2004). In Fiorio et al. (2022), the placebo procedure may have shifted movement control from feedback to feedforward processes, even with an increasing level of difficulty of the task.

This evidence has the twofold impact of expanding our knowledge on placebo-induced effects on an as-yet-unexplored motor function (i.e., goal-directed movement), as well as paving the way for expectancy-based strategies to boost performance in goal-directed movements.

The placebo effect on visuo-motor learning of fingers sequences

Another key component of human motor functions is motor learning, especially motor skill learning. Many activities of daily life, such as cooking, writing, and playing a musical instrument, are acquired through repeated practice, through which isolated movements are converted into well-performed skills. During this learning process, motor execution acquires speed and precision over time (Dayan & Cohen, 2011; Diedrichsen & Kornysheva, 2015; Nissen & Bullemer, 1987; Perez et al., 2007; Villa-Sánchez et al., 2021; Wolpert et al., 2011). A recent study explored the possibility to improve motor skill learning by means of positive expectations. In the attempt to guarantee for experimental control, the serial reaction time task (SRTT) was used to assess the acquisition of motor skill (Villa-Sánchez et al., 2021). In this task, a visual stimulus appears in one of four positions on a PC monitor and the participant is asked to press a key corresponding to the position of the visual stimulus with one of four fingers as fast and accurately as possible. Participants typically become faster and more accurate with practice, thus indicating motor learning. Crucially, unbeknown to the participants, a deterministic sequence was hidden between blocks of random positions. Thus, by measuring the performance on the sequence and random trials both sequence-specific (skill) learning and general motor learning could be assessed. Since motor learning impinges upon the physical features of movement as well as cognitive functions, like attention – especially in the first phase of skills acquisition (Doyon et al., 2003; Janacsek & Nemeth, 2012; Kaufman et al., 2010) – the role of two types of placebos, one motor-related and one cognitive-related, was tackled. For the motor-related placebo intervention, TENS was applied to the body part involved in the motor task (i.e., the hand), accompanied by verbal suggestion that it could enhance execution of movement. For the cognitive-related placebo, transcranial direct current stimulation (tDCS) was applied to the forehead, accompanied by the verbal suggestion that it could boost attention and concentration. Unbeknown to the participants, the two interventions were inert (sham). Results showed that motor-related placebo could enhance general motor performance on the SRTT. This improvement, however, was not specific for the sequence trials, as it was present also in the random trials. Hence, it appears that the placebo-TENS generally improved response selection without affecting sequence-specific learning. The placebo-tDCS did not affect motor performance but was able to reduce the subjective perception of fatigue at both the mental and physical level. This finding hints at a potential beneficial impact of placebo-tDCS to aid perception of fatigue in contexts in which movements are repeated over a prolonged period of time and cognitive demand is high, like, for example, motor training or motor rehabilitation programs. Overall, this study indicates that motor- and cognitive-related placebos differently shape motor performance and perceived fatiguability on a repeated motor task (Villa-Sánchez et al., 2021).

The placebo effect on gross motor control of the whole body and of the lower limbs

Differently from fine and localised movements, whole-body performance mainly implies a gross motor control, that is the ability to perform large, broad movements (such as lifting a leg or any other total body/multi-limb movements), which requires adequate coordination and function of bones, nerves, and muscles. Moreover, whereas performance gains in gross motor tasks are mostly assessed using outcome measures such as scores, number of successful trials, etc., performance in fine motor tasks is usually measured by kinematic or biophysical measures such as movement or force variability or submovements.

The placebo effect on leg extension

Much of the research on placebos and motor performance falls under the domain of gross movements requiring a synergistic coordination of different body districts, especially in the field of sports. However, findings drawn from experimental laboratory conditions on healthy individuals point to a role of placebos, even for more specific motor tasks involving lower-limb movements. One example of this is the leg-extension exercise, a type of strength-training exercise engaging quadriceps muscles, which is performed in a seated position and consists of raising a roller pad by extending the knee whilst keeping the torso and back firmly pressed against the back pad, without allowing the hips or buttocks to lift off the seat, and then returning back to the starting position (Phillips, 1997).

In one study, Pollo et al. (2008) tested the effects of an ergogenic placebo on the performance of the quadriceps muscles assessed through leg extension. In a first experiment, the administration of a placebo accompanied by positive verbal suggestions that it was caffeine at high dose resulted in a significant increase in mean muscle work, though without a decrease in perceived muscle fatigue. In a second experiment, a non-pharmacological preconditioning procedure was employed, whereby placebo caffeine was administered twice in two different sessions in each of which the weight to be lifted with the quadriceps was surreptitiously reduced to strengthen participants' expectations about the force-enhancing properties of the "ergogenic agent". Following this conditioning procedure, the load was restored to the original weight, and the same placebo was administered to test its effects on muscle work and fatigue. Compared to the first experiment, participants showed a stronger placebo effect with regards to both of these outcome measures (i.e., increase in muscle work and decrease in perceived muscular fatigue), suggesting how learning mechanisms play a crucial role in reinforcing the magnitude of the placebo response, especially with regard to fatigue perception. Overall, the findings from both experiments confirm the involvement of a central mechanism of a top-down modulation of muscle fatigue, thus corroborating the line of thinking positing the involvement of central components in muscle performance.

The placebo effect on balance control

A stable and upright stance is needed in many daily life activities and is a fundamental requisite in the prevention of falls. Human stance is a dynamic rather than a static phenomenon (Boyas et al., 2013; Günther et al., 2009), characterised by small instabilities called body sways. Controlling posture through balance requires a complex organisation and interaction between motor coordination and sensory systems, such as the somatosensory, vestibular and visual systems (Horak, 1997; Peterka & Loughlin, 2004). The corticospinal system plays an important role in controlling standing balance (Obata et al., 2009; Tokuno et al., 2009). Crucially, the placebo effect in the motor domain increases the excitability of the corticospinal system (Fiorio et al., 2014), thus giving neurophysiological support to the potential link between the placebo effect and balance control. Starting from this evidence, one study tested the possibility of improving balance control in healthy individuals by means of positive expectations induced through a placebo procedure (Horak, 1997). Balance control was tested with a single-leg stance task in which participants stood as steadily as possible on their dominant leg. During the task, an accelerometer attached to the participants' leg allowed the measurement of body sways in different directions. In an experimental group, placebo-TENS was applied on the leg, together with verbal instructions on its effectiveness in improving balance. Results showed that placebo-TENS induced an overall decrease of body sways, hinting at better postural control (Villa-Sánchez et al., 2019). The improvement of balance was found not only at a general level, i.e., in the three-dimensional space, but also more specifically in the anterior-posterior plane, while no effect was found in the medio-lateral direction. This specific pattern could indicate that the placebo group developed a specific postural strategy, based on the ankle, to maintain the body aligned to the upright position.

Improving balance through a placebo procedure can have a beneficial impact on gait disorders in which the pharmacological treatment is often ineffective. Translational relevance of this study could be found also in clinical populations (e.g., Parkinson's disease) and in the elderly, in which balance disturbances increase the risk of falls with a consequent negative impact on the quality of life. Future research should clarify whether the improvement in balance control obtained with a placebo procedure could be comparable to that obtained with non-invasive stimulation of the cerebellum (Emadi Andani et al., 2020).

Conclusions

The evidence here reported represents a key addition to the already abundant literature on the power of placebo effects in motor performance. Indeed, recent experimental studies are not limited to well-trained athletes but extend to untrained, naïve healthy participants who are tested under controlled laboratory conditions during the execution of simple motor tasks. This shift in the context of investigation from areas in which the motor placebo effect is already well-established (i.e., sports and the clinical context) to controlled laboratory experiments has a twofold implication. On the one hand, it enables a more targeted investigation of movements that are not only performed with the whole body, as in sports, but also the ones that are performed with a single or restricted muscle group. In fact, the role of placebos also extends to more fine and localised movements, such as the abduction or flexion of the finger and the arm or extension of the leg. This, in turn, opens the possibility to conduct precise neurophysiological investigations and observe whether the effects can be detected in the complex neural circuitry subtending the cognitive control of movements, such as the corticospinal system, and the readiness potential. In a circular fashion, this basic approach may be the prelude to a more targeted translation of the findings back to clinical and sports contexts.

References

Benedetti, F., Pollo, A., & Colloca, L. (2007). Opioid-mediated placebo responses boost pain endurance and physical performance: Is it doping in sport competitions? *Journal of Neuroscience, 27*(44), 11934–11939.

Bottoms, L., Buscombe, R., & Nicholettos, A. (2014). The placebo and nocebo effects on peak minute power during incremental arm crank ergometry. *European Journal of Sport Science, 14*(4), 362–367.

Boyas, S., Hajj, M., & Bilodeau, M. (2013). Influence of ankle plantarflexor fatigue on postural sway, lower limb articular angles, and postural strategies during unipedal quiet standing. *Gait & Posture, 37*(4), 547–551.

Dayan, E., & Cohen, L. G. (2011). Neuroplasticity subserving motor skill learning. *Neuron, 72*(3), 443–454.

Desmurget, M., & Grafton, S. (2000). Forward modeling allows feedback control for fast reaching movements. *Trends in Cognitive Sciences, 4*(11), 423–431.

Diedrichsen, J., & Kornysheva, K. (2015). Motor skill learning between selection and execution. *Trends in Cognitive Sciences, 19*(4), 227–233.

Doyon, J., Penhune, V., & Ungerleider, L. G. (2003). Distinct contribution of the cortico-striatal and cortico-cerebellar systems to motor skill learning. *Neuropsychologia, 41*(3), 252–262.

Emadi Andani, M., Villa-Sánchez, B., Raneri, F., Dametto, S., Tinazzi, M., & Fiorio, M. (2020). Cathodal cerebellar tDCS combined with visual feedback improves balance control. *The Cerebellum, 19*, 812–823.

Fiorio, M., Emadi Andani, M., Marotta, A., Classen, J., & Tinazzi, M. (2014). Placebo-induced changes in excitatory and inhibitory corticospinal circuits during motor performance. *Journal of Neuroscience, 34*(11), 3993–4005.

Fiorio, M., Villa-Sánchez, B., Rossignati, F., & Emadi Andani, M. (2022). The placebo effect shortens movement time in goal-directed movements. *Scientific Reports, 12*(1), 19567.

Fitts, P. M. (1954). The information capacity of the human motor system in controlling the amplitude of movement. *Journal of Experimental Psychology, 47*(6), 381.

Günther, M., Grimmer, S., Siebert, T., & Blickhan, R. (2009). All leg joints contribute to quiet human stance: A mechanical analysis. *Journal of Biomechanics, 42*(16), 2739–2746.

Horak, F. B. (1997). Clinical assessment of balance disorders. *Gait & Posture, 6*(1), 76–84.

Hurst, P., Schipof-Godart, L., Szabo, A., Raglin, J., Hettinga, F., Roelands, B., Lane, A., Foad, A., Coleman, D., & Beedie, C. (2020). The placebo and nocebo effect on sports performance: A systematic review. *European Journal of Sport Science, 20*(3), 279–292.

Janacsek, K., & Nemeth, D. (2012). Predicting the future: From implicit learning to consolidation. *International Journal of Psychophysiology, 83*(2), 213–221.

Kato, K., Muraoka, T., Higuchi, T., Mizuguchi, N., & Kanosue, K. (2014). Interaction between simultaneous contraction and relaxation in different limbs. *Experimental Brain Research, 232*, 181–189.

Kaufman, S. B., DeYoung, C. G., Gray, J. R., Jiménez, L., Brown, J., & Mackintosh, N. (2010). Implicit learning as an ability. *Cognition, 116*(3), 321–340.

Lidstone, S. C., Schulzer, M., Dinelle, K., Mak, E., Sossi, V., Ruth, T. J., de la Fuente-Fernández, R., Phillips, A. G., & Stoessl, A. J. (2010). Effects of expectation on placebo-induced dopamine release in Parkinson disease. *Archives of General Psychiatry, 67*(8), 857–865.

Nissen, M. J., & Bullemer, P. (1987). Attentional requirements of learning: Evidence from performance measures. *Cognitive Psychology, 19*(1), 1–32.

Obata, H., Sekiguchi, H., Nakazawa, K., & Ohtsuki, T. (2009). Enhanced excitability of the corticospinal pathway of the ankle extensor and flexor muscles during standing in humans. *Experimental Brain Research, 197*, 207–213.

Perez, M. A., Wise, S. P., Willingham, D. T., & Cohen, L. G. (2007). Neurophysiological mechanisms involved in transfer of procedural knowledge. *Journal of Neuroscience, 27*(5), 1045–1053.

Peterka, R. J., & Loughlin, P. J. (2004). Dynamic regulation of sensorimotor integration in human postural control. *Journal of Neurophysiology, 91*(1), 410–423.

Phillips, N. (1997). Essentials of strength training and conditioning. *Physiotherapy, 83*(1).

Piedimonte, A., Benedetti, F., & Carlino, E. (2015). Placebo-induced decrease in fatigue: Evidence for a central action on the preparatory phase of movement. *European Journal of Neuroscience, 41*(4), 492–497.

Pollo, A., Carlino, E., & Benedetti, F. (2008). The top-down influence of ergogenic placebos on muscle work and fatigue. *European Journal of Neuroscience, 28*(2), 379–388.

Rossettini, G., Emadi Andani, M., Dalla Negra, F., Testa, M., Tinazzi, M., & Fiorio, M. (2018). The placebo effect in the motor domain is differently modulated by the external and internal focus of attention. *Scientific Reports, 8*(1), 1–14.

Seidler, R. D., Noll, D. C., & Thiers, G. (2004). Feedforward and feedback processes in motor control. *NeuroImage, 22*(4), 1775–1783.

Spraker, M. B., Corcos, D. M., & Vaillancourt, D. E. (2009). Cortical and subcortical mechanisms for precisely controlled force generation and force relaxation. *Cerebral Cortex, 19*(11), 2640–2650.

Tokuno, C., Taube, W., & Cresswell, A. (2009). An enhanced level of motor cortical excitability during the control of human standing. *Acta Physiologica, 195*(3), 385–395.

Villa-Sánchez, B., Emadi Andani, M., Cesari, P., & Fiorio, M. (2021). The effect of motor and cognitive placebos on the serial reaction time task. *European Journal of Neuroscience, 53*(8), 2655–2668.

Villa-Sánchez, B., Emadi Andani, M., Menegaldo, G., Tinazzi, M., & Fiorio, M. (2019). Positive verbal suggestion optimizes postural control. *Scientific Reports, 9*(1), 1–10.

Wolpert, D. M., Diedrichsen, J., & Flanagan, J. R. (2011). Principles of sensorimotor learning. *Nature Reviews Neuroscience, 12*(12), 739–751.

11

HOW DO I USE PLACEBO EFFECTS TO IMPROVE MY INTERVENTIONS?

Harnessing knowledge of placebo effects to maximise the effectiveness of interventions in sport

Andrew M. Lane, Ross Cloak, and Tracey J. Devonport

Introduction

A placebo effect is a positive effect which cannot be attributed to active ingredients in the treatment (Beedie et al., 2018; Beedie et al., 2020; Marticorena et al., 2021). A nocebo effect is the opposite; this is where an intervention was conducted, but beliefs in the likely effects were sufficiently negative to explain a lack of improvement or drop in performance. Beedie et al. (2018, 2020) have written extensively on the mechanism of placebo effects, calling for work to understand the neurobiological mechanisms. Beedie et al. (2020) discuss the impact of conditioning and expectancies through which people ascribe positive or negative beliefs ahead of, during, and following receipt of a treatment, and it is logical to assume that such beliefs will follow through to behaviour. Practitioners can influence an individual's expectations about the effects of a treatment for better or for worse. This is dependent on how the treatment is described, including anticipated outcomes. Have you ever noticed that sports energy gels with caffeine are more expensive than energy gels without caffeine? Is it that people are willing to pay that little bit more for what they believe to be the active ingredient in helping to combat sensations of fatigue. The notion is that people are using the price of the product as a proxy for how good it is, and the reason why it might be more effective is that it strengthens beliefs.

Practitioners work with clients who wish to achieve their goals (Lane, 2018; Lane et al., 2014; Lochbaum, Sherburn, et al., 2022; Lochbaum, Stoner, et al., 2022), whether that is a professional athlete striving to achieve an Olympic medal, a recreational athlete personal best, in fact any performance-related goal. The same is true in exercise, where people wish to get fitter, lose weight, feel healthier and use treatments to help achieve this. If placebo effects

DOI: 10.4324/9781003229001-11

have additional benefits, then it makes sense for practitioners to facilitate positive beliefs (expectancies) in clients before they start to use a treatment. If this is achieved, then the beliefs themselves not only have direct effects, but can increase the effectiveness of the treatment (Bandura, 2018; Bandura et al., 1999; Lochbaum, Sherburn, et al., 2022). We think that practitioners should assess and develop beliefs, and thereby treat beliefs as an active component of the treatment (Roelands & Hurst, 2020; Smith et al., 2021). In this chapter, we discuss issues related to the use of placebo effects in applied work. The three authors are all practitioners and draw upon nearly 30 years of experience of working in applied & exercise sports science. Where possible, we cite research to support our ideas, but the absence of specific research that looks at the incremental value of beliefs means that we also speculate on the basis of logic. As highlighted recently (Roelands & Hurst, 2020), theory develops via evidence and proposals, and therefore one aim of our chapter is to encourage future researchers to identify and test the effects of placebo/nocebo beliefs in their work.

Starting with an example… What if you were working with a boxer and a treatment appears to work but is a placebo?

We will start the discussion via the use of an example to help us keep our discussion grounded in real-world scenarios. Imagine the scene: You are a sports scientist working with a combat sport athlete in preparation for a career defining contest (Matthews et al., 2019; Morton et al., 2010; Smith et al., 2022), a scenario all three authors of its chapter have experienced. You have 12 weeks to plan the programme and have many challenges to consider in preparing the athlete. This includes their dropping multiple kilograms to make weight while retaining or even gaining strength, all the time ensuring they remain highly confident in being able to perform on the night of the fight. These factors will work interactively rather than in isolation (Matthews et al., 2019; Morton et al., 2010). For example, an athlete's confidence should increase if they get stronger, feel prepared, and be close to competition weight (Smith et al., 2022). The athlete follows a treatment designed to improve performance which comprises many different techniques. If the athlete feels more confident, performs to their ability, and wins the contest, the practitioner is seen as effective by association. This association is strengthened if the athlete values the relationship with the source of the information. For example, advice and the importance of such advice when making weight in Taekwondo has a greater influence over beliefs when provided by the coach or by other athletes than when provided by nutritionists or doctors (Smith et al., 2022). For practitioners, this highlights the importance of having the support of the coach, and that the messages given are consistent.

In the scenario presented above, we cannot really know the extent to which the treatment contributed to improved performance. This is normal; the researchers did not set out to assess the contribution of belief effects to the success of the work. A missing ingredient from much research is the identification and quantification of such active, but often-hidden components of the treatment, and without such knowledge we cannot know exactly why it worked. Superstitions in sport work in this way, for example players wear their lucky socks, but we know there are no physical qualities in the lucky socks that lead to improved performance over and above other socks. But we do know that when the person wears their lucky socks, they feel more confident, which in turn leads to better performance. Similar logic to the lucky socks can apply when a practitioner suggests using a treatment, but in either case any effect could be a placebo effect. Further, it is possible that if the athlete's performance is poor, and the treatment is criticised for being ineffective, this could be ascribed to a nocebo effect, where negative beliefs and expectations in following the treatment are influential. From a practitioner perspective, having the placebo effect on your side is favourable. Therefore, with this point in mind, we will pick a treatment a practitioner might typically use, for illustrative purposes, and we look at how placebo effects might help athletes perform better and a nocebo effect might worsen performance.

Returning to our combat sport athlete seeking to improve performance, we might suggest using psychological skills training (PST). A technique commonly used in preparing athletes for competition is the psychological skill of imagery. Imagery is where an individual mentally pictures an activity using all the senses (sight, sound, feel, and taste; Pearson, 2019; Simonsmeier et al., 2021). The athlete uses imagery to regulate their anxiety and strengthen confidence to execute the fight plan (Kasiri et al., 2017). The athlete's performance starts improving, and they report increased confidence. You also notice that they are much closer to their fighting weight, scores on fitness tests are better, and they are generally calmer and happier. The imagery treatment is the only meaningful change to previous training and the boxer is very pleased. In this example, imagery is the new treatment, and looks like it is working, but the mechanism through which performance is improving could be attributed to other factors.

In the example above, imagery appeared to be successful. However, as we did not assess the mechanisms through which success was achieved it could have been due to factors that were not directly associated with the treatment. It could be that a change in diet helped improve the quality of training, which, in turn, also helped trim weight and so nutritional changes are playing an important part. What does the practitioner do at this junction? Do they allow the athlete to continue to believe the positive effects being experienced are directly related to using imagery, even if theory on how imagery might help performance does not directly support this assumption? Do they inform the athlete, which could have a counterproductive effect, leading to uncertainty and doubt (as they do not know why performance is improving, they might believe that just as good performance suddenly came around, then so could poor performance).

In such a scenario it is worthwhile for professional development of the practitioner to interrogate the mechanisms of the improved performance.

Placebo effects and the practitioner – are positive effects due to persuasive educational methods?

We propose that placebo effects cover all disciplines and aspects of the sport sciences (Beedie et al., 2018). The type of treatment sports scientists use include prescribing training programmes, using heart rate to monitor training intensity, or analysing technique, whereas sport and exercise psychologists might encourage using psychological skills such as imagery, self-talk, or goal-setting which encourage changes in the way people think or use a strategy such as listening to music to regulate emotions. The treatment is typically delivered by a practitioner in the form of a consultation and any associated placebo effect is influenced by a number of factors, for example the perceived status of the practitioner to the athlete, the athlete's knowledge and experience, and the persuasiveness with which the treatment is delivered. We know that there are practitioner effects in the applied and medical sciences; recent research discussed the importance of regulating client's emotions, building on a wealth of evidence that empathy is a key practitioner skill and as such being able to read emotions is useful (Geers et al., 2021; Lane, 2020). Further, recent research found that treatments delivered online by former Olympian Michael Johnson were associated with stronger confidence, adaptive emotions, greater effort, and beliefs that the treatment helped mental preparation when compared with individuals not receiving the treatment (Lane et al., 2021; Lane et al., 2016).

Persuasive treatment can also be delivered via the methods used by practitioners to promote the treatments they use. A practitioner should, of course, suggest a treatment knowing that it should have a positive effect and knowing the reasons why it will likely work. The nutritional ergogenic aids industry has grown exponentially with popular products, including beetroot, protein, caffeine, and sports drinks among others. The industry has worked with sports scientists to test the efficacy of their products, with varying degrees of success. It is fair to say that it is common to see sports scientists endorse such products. In theory, athletes and exercisers will only pay for a product if they believe it will work. But 'work' speaks to more than just the biochemistry or substance of the product. A recent example of this is the use of creatine monohydrate (one of the most researched ergogenic aids in sports; Aguiar et al., 2022), for which evidence indicates that athletes who ingested creatine prior to a workout, as well as those who simply believed they had ingested creatine, performed significantly better resistance exercise to exhaustion then when under control conditions. Arguing the efficacy of acute supplementation may have more to do with the belief one attributes to it working rather than any physiological mechanism (Aguiar et al., 2022).

A placebo effect is likely to be part of a treatment as there is insufficient evidence to prescribe a dose-response effect

One issue that complicates matters is the relative strength of evidence in support of the effects of a treatment. With reference to our combat sport example, we cannot say imagery will improve performance with 100% confidence. Further, the evidence available in support of the effectiveness of treatments is rarely strong enough to be able to report a dose-response effect (Beedie et al., 2018; Hurst et al., 2020). So when working with an athlete, how much imagery we encourage them to use is unclear. It becomes plausible to think that if the athlete strongly believes doing imagery will work, then they might practice more seriously with greater focus and via this approach accrue more benefit than someone who believes it might not work. Therefore, we suggest practitioners should consider using the positive effects of a placebo. If we wanted supporting evidence that self-confidence helps athletes perform better, then a recent systematic review showed a positive relationship to performance (Lochbaum, Sherburn, et al., 2022). Practitioners working to raise confidence to improve performance must accept that if performance increases hugely then it's likely some other factors are at play (Beedie et al., 2020). A similar argument can be made for many variables – when the data are scrutinised researchers usually suggest that the rigour used in the research is not sufficiently strong enough to be confident that variable A causes changes in variable B (Beedie et al., 2020).

As self-report is often the best, and sometimes the only, method to identify and quantify a psychological process, there will always be a degree of error that is difficult to explain (Nisbett & Wilson, 1977). When presented with an item such a 'how anxious do you feel?' and being asked to rate that on an arbitrary scale, such as 0 = not at all to 4 = very much so, an individual scans their feeling. The subsequent number they use is an estimate of their feelings. The use of self-report in construct measurement is a key feature of the challenge to find a rigorous design to show causation. Self-report is used in many studies, from psychological constructs of mood, emotion, self-confidence, motivation etc, to supposedly physiological constructs such as perceived exertion. In other contexts, self-report is used by nutritionists for diet diaries or in skill acquisition via estimating hours of practice. Self-report will always provide an estimate as the accuracy of memory and the emotional state at the time of recall are influential (Terry et al., 2005).

A second feature is the rigour of the research design (Beedie et al., 2020; Lane et al., 2021; Lane et al., 2016). Control groups are needed to account for the effects of a placebo. The mechanisms through which a placebo could work are likely to be around raised expectancy beliefs and self-efficacy. The psychological investment in taking a treatment will be stronger in a real-world setting where the individual is actively striving to achieve a goal. And so, people take trying to achieve the task more seriously and place more hope in the treatment working. In experimental studies, arguably people do not take goal achievement so seriously, and, as such, a treatment to help goal striving is of less importance. Research has found people placebo themselves (Beedie, 2007), that is, they took a performance-enhancing ergogenic that they strongly believed worked, only later to find out it was not. Therefore, in summary, the role of placebo beliefs versus nocebo beliefs is not well understood, but self-efficacy beliefs do influence performance, and so it seems appropriate to raise beliefs in most cases to improve the chances that a treatment might work. We cover the ethics of positively encouraging use of a treatment in the next section.

Is it ethical to prescribe a treatment when its effectiveness might be due to a belief effect?

A clear ethical code of practice is to not falsify treatments. If the practitioner is truly unsure that the treatment will work, does not know the proposed mechanics through which it works, and even suspects that it could be detrimental or harmful, then the risk of using that treatment is too great, and, indeed, unethical. We argue that practitioners should use placebo effects to provide added value to using a treatment where there should be clear theoretical reasons, mechanisms of effect identified, and some supporting evidence. We argue that practitioners should aim to harness, with harness being a carefully chosen term, the mechanisms underlying placebo effects. We argue that research is needed to identify the strength of placebo effects and how they relate to the actual treatment individual is using. The absence of such research has spawned, what we feel is a worse scenario, where people follow a treatment where there is no real strong effect, and the mechanisms are not adequately explained (perhaps hoping for a placebo effect?).

In terms of why a practitioner might wish to enhance beliefs in order to catalyse a placebo effect, we have drawn on research that suggests that the quality of the practitioner is an active ingredient in that treatment. Evidence from medical consultations points to positive effects for consultants with good interpersonal skills (Geers et al., 2021). The practitioner might be effective by improving mood, even though this might not be the intended effect; that is, for example, the client might be seeking a consultation to enable them to run a marathon faster. However, feeling better and less anxious could lead to better quality sleep, less stress, even less muscle tension, and via the collective effects of these discrete processes experience better-quality training, better recovery, and therefore better adaptations, leading to better performance. Consistent with recent suggestions from clinical practice we believe that the practitioner should be open to the possible effects of placebo or nocebo beliefs and inform the client accordingly (Evers et al., 2021a, 2021b). We believe that this is an ethical approach to take as it does not seek to hide the benefits of beliefs.

Self-efficacy estimates in the effectiveness of the intervention as a construct to assess placebo beliefs

Self-efficacy theory (Bandura, 2018; Bandura et al., 1999) could offer a theoretical framework through which beliefs are strengthened. A recent systematic review indicated the benefits of self-confidence on performance (Lochbaum, Sherburn, et al., 2022; Lochbaum, Stoner, et al., 2022). As proposed by self-efficacy theory, when efficacy increases there is increased commitment and persistence in the face of setbacks. A key point here is that there needs to be improved performance or perceived improvements in performance. Perceived improvement is common in endurance performance where athletes report running at the same pace to be easier the more frequently they do it, and so confidence increases. Self-efficacy is an ecumenical psychological process in which information from all sources is integrated via cognitive processes. And therefore, for example, it allows an understanding of the extent to which changes in nutrition might influence self-efficacy via creating beliefs that, for example, the fighting weight can be made, and the strength retained, while still being able to train adequately and nutritionally fuelled, which are all common fears for combat sport participants. If the treatment to improve beliefs regarding altering nutrition is based on a placebo, that is, there is no real reason only beliefs, but the boxer gains confidence, perceives greater self-control, and loses weight by having fewer episodes of emotional eating; then arguably the treatment is worth continuing (Figure 11.1).

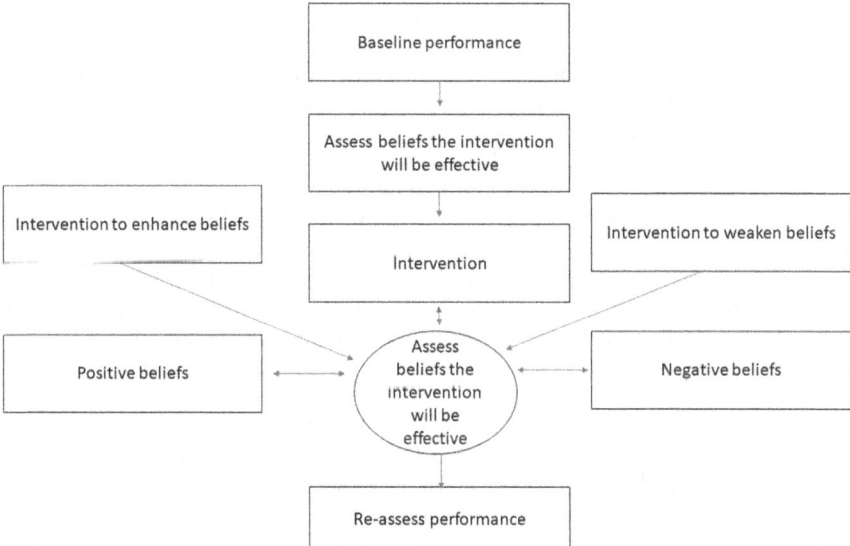

FIGURE 11.1 Proposed model of working with beliefs effects when delivering interventions.

Conclusions

We think that, in practice, most practitioners carry on using suggested interventions, recognising that these carry indirect benefits. However, if a practitioner follows the science strictly, then they should acknowledge that the positive effects could be a placebo effect. There are tensions that arise from trying to apply science to practice, in that the strength of (publicly available) evidence creates the possibility, as with this illustrative example, that a placebo effect might underlie some of the positive effects of treatments. A key point to make at the start when working with clients is that practitioners apply scientific theory and evidence in seeking to improve performance or help well-being, and that placebo effects could contribute to many positive effects in their work.

References

Aguiar, M. S., Pereira, R., Koch, A. J., & Machado, M. (2022). Psychological effect of acute creatine pre-workout supplementation induces performance improvement in resistance exercise. *Research in Sports Medicine*, 1–12.

Bandura, A. (2018). Toward a psychology of human agency: Pathways and reflections. *Perspectives on Psychological Science*, *13*(2), 130–136.

Bandura, A., Freeman, W. H., & Lightsey, R. (1999). Self-efficacy: The exercise of control. *Journal of Cognitive Psychotherapy*, *13*(2), 158-166.

Beedie, C. (2007). Placebo effects in competitive sport: Qualitative data. *Journal of Sports Science and Medicine*, *6*(1), 21.

Beedie, C., Benedetti, F., Barbiani, D., Camerone, E., Cohen, E., Coleman, D., Davis, A., Elsworth-Edelsten, C., Flowers, E., & Foad, A. (2018). Consensus statement on placebo effects in sports and exercise: The need for conceptual clarity, methodological rigour, and the elucidation of neurobiological mechanisms. *European Journal of Sport Science*, *18*(10), 1383–1389.

Beedie, C., Benedetti, F., Barbiani, D., Camerone, E., Lindheimer, J., & Roelands, B. (2020). Incorporating methods and findings from neuroscience to better understand placebo and nocebo effects in sport. *European Journal of Sport Science*, *20*(3), 313–325.

Evers, A. W., Colloca, L., Blease, C., Gaab, J., Jensen, K. B., Atlas, L. Y., Beedie, C. J., Benedetti, F., Bingel, U., & Büchel, C. (2021a). "Consensus on placebo and nocebo effects connects science with practice:" Reply to "questioning the consensus on placebo and nocebo effects". *Psychotherapy and Psychosomatics*, *90*(3), 213–214.

Evers, A. W., Colloca, L., Blease, C., Gaab, J., Jensen, K. B., Atlas, L. Y., Beedie, C. J., Benedetti, F., Bingel, U., & Büchel, C. (2021b). What should clinicians tell patients about placebo and nocebo effects? Practical considerations based on expert consensus. *Psychotherapy and Psychosomatics*, *90*(1), 49–56.

Geers, A. L., Faasse, K., Guevarra, D. A., Clemens, K. S., Helfer, S. G., & Colagiuri, B. (2021). Affect and emotions in placebo and nocebo effects: What do we know so far?. *Social and Personality Psychology Compass*, *15*(1), e12575. https://doi.org/10.1111/spc3.12575

Hurst, P., Schipof-Godart, L., Szabo, A., Raglin, J., Hettinga, F., Roelands, B., Lane, A., Foad, A., Coleman, D., & Beedie, C. (2020). The placebo and nocebo effect on sports performance: A systematic review. *European Journal of Sport Science, 20*(3), 279–292.

Kasiri, S., Fookes, C., Sridharan, S., & Morgan, S. (2017). Fine-grained action recognition of boxing punches from depth imagery. *Computer Vision and Image Understanding, 159*, 143–153.

Lane, A. (2018). From idea to impact: Sharing your work and getting it noticed. *Psychreg Journal of Psychology, 2*(1), 1–5.

Lane, A. M. (2020). Emotion and emotion regulation from the perspective of the practitioner. In Ruiz, M. C., & Robazza, C. (Eds.). *Feelings in sport: theory, research, and practical implications for performance and well-being* (pp. 187–198). Routledge.

Lane, A. M., Beedie, C. J., Devonport, T. J., & Friesen, A. P. (2021). Considerations of control groups: Comparing active-control with no treatment for examining the effects of brief intervention. *Sports, 9*(11), 156.

Lane, A. M., Godfrey, R. J., Loosemore, M., & Whyte, G. P. (2014). *Case studies in sport science and medicine.* CreateSpace.

Lane, A. M., Totterdell, P., MacDonald, I., Devonport, T. J., Friesen, A. P., Beedie, C. J., Stanley, D., & Nevill, A. (2016). Brief online training enhances competitive performance: Findings of the BBC Lab UK psychological skills intervention study. *Frontiers in Psychology, 7*, 413.

Lochbaum, M., Sherburn, M., Sisneros, C., Cooper, S., Lane, A. M., & Terry, P. C. (2022). Revisiting the Self-Confidence and Sport Performance Relationship: A Systematic Review with Meta-Analysis. *International Journal of Environmental Research and Public Health, 19*(11), 6381.

Lochbaum, M., Stoner, E., Hefner, T., Cooper, S., Lane, A. M., & Terry, P. C. (2022). Sport psychology and performance meta-analyses: A systematic review of the literature. *PLoS One, 17*(2), e0263408.

Marticorena, F. M., Carvalho, A., de Oliveira, L. F., Dolan, E., Gualano, B., Swinton, P., & Saunders, B. (2021). Nonplacebo controls to determine the magnitude of ergogenic interventions: A systematic review and meta-analysis. *Medicine and Science in Sports and Exercise, 53*(8), 1766–1777.

Matthews, J. J., Stanhope, E. N., Godwin, M. S., Holmes, M. E., & Artioli, G. G. (2019). The magnitude of rapid weight loss and rapid weight gain in combat sport athletes preparing for competition: A systematic review. *International Journal of Sport Nutrition and Exercise Metabolism, 29*(4), 441–452.

Morton, J. P., Robertson, C., & Sutton, L. (2010). Making the weight: A case study from professional boxing. *International Journal of Sport Nutrition and Exercise Metabolism, 20*(1), 80–85.

Nisbett, R. E., & Wilson, T. D. (1977). Telling more than we can know: Verbal reports on mental processes. *Psychological Review, 84*(3), 231.

Pearson, J. (2019). The human imagination: The cognitive neuroscience of visual mental imagery. *Nature Reviews Neuroscience, 20*(10), 624–634.

Roelands, B., & Hurst, P. (2020). The placebo effect in sport: How practitioners can inject words to improve performance. *International Journal of Sports Physiology and Performance, 15*(6), 765–766.

Simonsmeier, B. A., Andronie, M., Buecker, S., & Frank, C. (2021). The effects of imagery interventions in sports: A meta-analysis. *International Review of Sport and Exercise Psychology, 14*(1), 186–207.

Smith, K. A., Naughton, R. J., Langan-Evans, C., & Lewis, K. (2022). "Horrible—but worth it": Exploring weight cutting practices, eating behaviors, and experiences of competitive female taekwon-do athletes. A mixed methods study. *Journal of Clinical Sport Psychology*, *1*(aop), 1–15.

Smith, K. A., Vennik, J., Morrison, L., Hughes, S., Steele, M., Tiwari, R., Bostock, J., Howick, J., Mallen, C., & Little, P. (2021). Harnessing placebo effects in primary care: Using the person-based approach to develop an online intervention to enhance practitioners' communication of clinical empathy and realistic optimism during consultations. *Frontiers in Pain Research*, *2*, 49. doi.org/10.3389/fpain.2021.721222

Terry, P. C., Stevens, M. J., & Lane, A. M. (2005). Influence of response time frame on mood assessment. *Anxiety, Stress, and Coping*, *18*(3), 279–285.

12

DO YOU HAVE TO LIE TO INDUCE PLACEBO EFFECTS?

The use of open label placebos in sport and exercise

Bryan Saunders, Felipe Miguel Marticorena, and Bruno Gualano

Introduction

Exercise performance can be modified via both placebo and nocebo effects (Hurst et al., 2020), with coaches and athletes seeking methods to optimise these placebo effects to maximise exercise performance. However, the use of deceptive placebo in practice is inherently fraught with ethical constraints and trust issues, meaning alternative methods must be employed in practice. This has led to the development of an alternative approach through which placebo effects might be generated, namely open-label placebo (OLP). This concept, also termed "honest placebo", consists of openly informing the individual that they are receiving an inert intervention (i.e., a placebo). Although apparently counterintuitive, since placebo effects are often believed to stem from the individual's belief that they are receiving an active treatment (Kaptchuk et al., 2010; Miller & Colloca, 2009) there is a growing body of evidence demonstrating the efficacy of this method in a clinical practice. While data in the sport and exercise sector remain scarce, preliminary evidence does exist with scope for further work and real-world application.

Open-label placebo

Evidence of placebo effects is now established in the sport and exercise literature (for reviews see: Beedie et al., 2018; Beedie & Foad, 2009; Hurst et al., 2020) and performance changes can be attributed to physiological responses to a placebo treatment (Benedetti et al., 2007; Finniss et al., 2010). It has been a longstanding belief that deceptive application of a placebo, namely communicating to the individual that they are receiving an active treatment,

DOI: 10.4324/9781003229001-12

i) Placebos are powerful

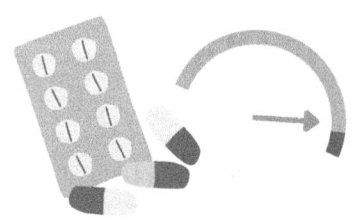

iii) Positive attitude

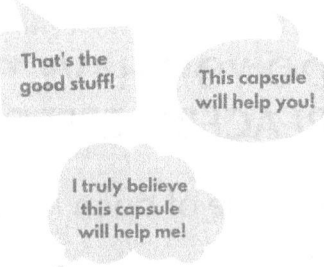

ii) Effects of conditioning

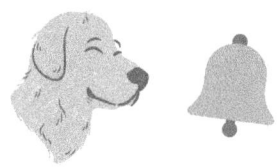

iv) Take the pills!

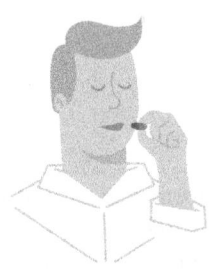

FIGURE 12.1 The four main discussion points to be discussed with the individual during the open-label placebo intervention, namely that i) placebo effects are powerful; ii) the body may automatically respond to taking placebo pills similar to Pavlov's dogs; iii) a positive attitude helps; and iv) taking the pills is a critical component.

is required to elicit placebo effects. However, OLP goes against the grain in actively and openly informing the individual that the treatment they are receiving is inert. Nonetheless, the way in which this information is delivered likely plays an important role in the subsequent outcomes. Were the information provided in a negative and unenthusiastic manner relating to the placebo, one would certainly not expect positive benefits, and a nocebo response may even be expected. If the information is provided more positively, then one might expect similarly positive outcomes. Indeed, in the original OLP studies by Ted Kaptchuk, the way in which information regarding the OLP is provided to patients appears to be positive (Kaptchuk et al., 2010), with four main discussion points to be discussed with the individual (Figure 12.1):

1. Placebo effects are powerful;
2. The body may automatically respond to taking placebo pills; similar to Pavlov's dogs who salivated when they heard a bell;

3. A positive attitude helps, but is not entirely necessary as the response may be automatic;
4. Taking the pills is a critical component.

Applying such a positive framing to the placebo would, in theory, optimise the chance of a positive response.

The concept of OLP is in direct contrast to the commonly held notion that deception and belief in a treatment is required to elicit beneficial effects, and clinical research into non-deceptive placebos has emphatically turned this notion on its head. Extensive data now shows that openly informing individuals that they are receiving a placebo treatment can lead to significant and clinically meaningful improvements in symptoms of a number of different conditions compared to no-treatment (or treatment-as-usual) controls, such as irritable bowel syndrome (Kaptchuk et al., 2010) chronic lower back pain (Grotle & Hagen, 2017), allergic rhinitis (Schaefer et al., 2016; Schaefer et al., 2018), depression (Kelley et al., 2012) and cancer-related fatigue (Hoenemeyer et al., 2018; Zhou et al., 2019). Conditioned OLP may also help to reduce the quantity of self-prescribed pain killers (opioids) required to treat pain in individuals following spinal surgery, as recently demonstrated by Flowers and colleagues (Flowers et al., 2021). These data demonstrate the potential role of OLP in controlling sensation of pain and fatigue in various clinical populations. This could have interesting implications for sport since pain can be a limiting factor to performance during exercise (Canestri et al., 2021; Khan et al., 2011), while reducing or delaying sensations of fatigue is the holy grail for athletes aiming for peak performance.

Open-label placebo in exercise

Evidence for OLP in exercise is in its infancy, with only three peer-reviewed studies to date directly having investigated this. Performance across these studies was measured via a 1-km cycling time-trial (Saunders et al., 2019), muscular performance using maximal voluntary contractions of the lower limbs (Swafford et al., 2019), and handgrip strength and peak oxygen consumption (VO_{2peak}) during incremental cycling (Rossow et al., 2019). While a small beneficial effect was shown for 1-km cycling, no other improvements in exercise performance were shown in these studies. While these data do not immediately appear overly supportive of OLP for exercise performance, the devil may be in the details. Indeed, with only a few studies available, it is necessary to understand what moderating factors may alter the efficacy of an OLP intervention.

Saunders et al. (2019) recruited 28 female cyclists to participate in a study in which participants underwent an acute open-placebo intervention or a control session. The open-placebo intervention consisted of a standardised presentation about placebo and open-placebo provided by a female physician wearing a lab coat prior to the exercise test. This presenter explained the concept of placebo, detailing evidence of placebo effects in clinical and sports settings, before explaining the concept of open-placebo, and demonstrating evidence in a clinical setting. The presentation ended with a 3-point system of how to benefit from open-placebo incorporating the 4-point system of Kaptchuk and colleagues (Kaptchuk et al., 2010) highlighting that the placebo effect is powerful, a positive attitude helps but is not necessary since the response may be automatic, and that taking the pills is a critical component for an effect to occur. After ingesting two red and white capsules, the participants were then required to wait 15 min for "the pills to work", during which time they could chat with the physician and ask questions. Thereafter, they were taken to the laboratory next door, where they performed a 1-km cycling time-trial with two researchers blinded to the intervention. The control session began with a 20-minute wait in the same room with the same physicians, during which time they could chat freely, before being taken to the lab for the same exercise test. Performance was significantly improved with the OLP compared to the control session, with a very small positive effect on performance (effect size, d = 0.16). The same authors have recently repeated their findings in both male and female cyclists using a 4-km cycling time-trial (Barreto et al., 2021 conference proceedings), with significant overall improvements in performance in a cohort of 54 cyclists (effect size, d = 0.18).

Swafford et al. (2019) informed 21 untrained participants that "clinical studies have shown that OLP treatments enhance function and minimize pain", though they were also told not to expect to feel any effects. The authors provided a blue capsule to participants as they considered this to have perceived calming effects according to a meta-analysis (De Craen et al., 1996). It is unclear whether these factors influenced performance, but no subsequent benefits of the intervention were shown.

Rossow et al. (2019) provided neutral and objective information to their participants regarding the OLP employed in their study using a standardised script. Specifically, they informed participants that they would receive a placebo that had no significant physiological effect and confirmed that they understood what a placebo was. They were then provided with the placebo pill, though no descriptive information was provided as to its appearance. Results were compared to a dishonest placebo, where participants were informed they were receiving a pre-workout supplement that may increase their exercise performance, and a control session consisting of the exercise tests only. No differences between any visit were shown for either handgrip strength or VO_{2peak}.

Key differences in how the information regarding OLP was delivered may explain, at least in part, some of the differences in results between studies. The power of OLP likely comes from the entire intervention, starting from the

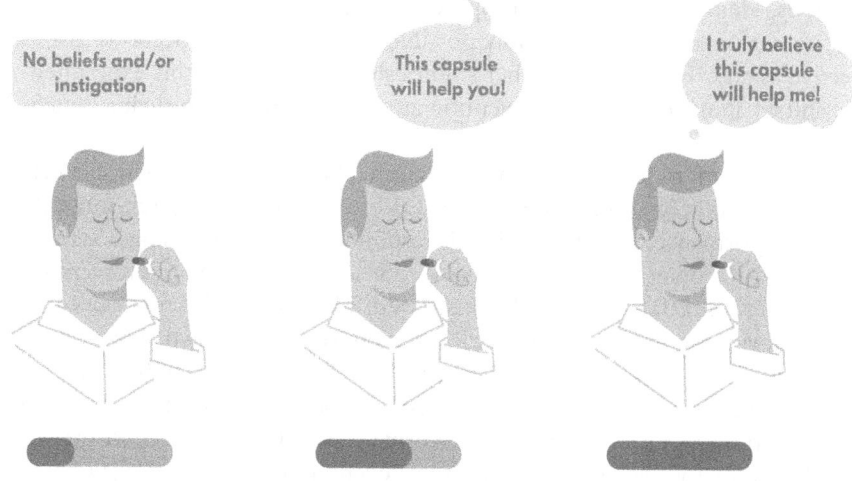

Intervention Effectiveness

FIGURE 12.2   The efficacy of the open-label placebo intervention may depend upon the information provided. If the evaluator provides little to no information, then a smaller response may be expected. Providing more information will likely increase the efficacy of the intervention, and if the participant themselves buys into this concept, then they can expect the greatest results.

attitude and behaviour of the researchers, to the way in which OLP is communicated to the individual (Davis et al., 2020), which will likely influence the individual's beliefs (Figure 12.2). The intervention by Saunders et al. (2019) was clearly designed to induce positive expectation in the intervention, and the authors even reported their intent in doing so. The information provided by Swafford et al. (2019) and Rossow et al. (2019) was more neutral, meaning participants were unlikely to have positive expectations regarding the intervention (Figure 12.2). Overall, these data indicate that positive expectation may form an integral component of any ergogenic improvement resulting from OLP, and this will stem from the manner in which the intervention is performed. This is somewhat supported by the systematic review of Hurst and colleagues (Hurst et al., 2020) which showed no effect of open-placebo on performance from balanced placebo designs (effect size, d = 0.08), which generally provide neutral information regarding the efficacy of the placebo session. Individual data from Saunders et al. (2019) also provide support for this argument, since all 4 individuals who worsened performed following OLP had some form of negative emotion relating to the intervention or their performance. Nonetheless, not all individuals who improved conveyed positive emotions, demonstrating the complex relationship between emotion and exercise performance. It is certainly possible that open-label nocebo is just as effective as an OLP, though further studies should determine this experimentally and what aspects of the intervention are most important to elicit a beneficial effect.

It is important to note that despite the overall beneficial performance effects shown by Saunders et al. (2019) of an OLP intervention on high-intensity cycling performance, not all individuals responded positively. Using a statistical method for determining individual response to a nutritional intervention (Swinton et al., 2018), four individuals were identified as having worsened their performance following the OLP intervention. It is known that nocebo effects can also moderate exercise performance (Hurst et al., 2020), with the size of these effects of similar magnitude to placebo effects, though in an unwanted direction (i.e., harmful to performance). If OLP is to be adopted as a viable and real-world strategy to improve exercise performance, it is important that the reasons behind why some individuals may experience worsened performance are determined so that these can be avoided as best as possible.

How does open-label placebo work?

Only one study to date has specifically measured potential mechanisms of OLP, although this was not in relation to exercise performance. Guevarra et al. (2020) measured the late positive potential, a neural biomarker of emotional distress, using electroencephalography to determine whether an OLP intervention could alter this psychobiological measure following a negative picture viewing task. The OLP reduced self-reported emotional distress and the late positive potential, demonstrating that OLP can generate measurable changes in psychobiology which can explain the impact of OLP on self-reported distress. This study is the first evidence to show that OLP effects are not just response bias but produce tangible mechanistic changes and physiological mechanisms through which subjective feeling are altered.

The placebo effect is a psychobiological phenomenon that can be attributed to several different mechanisms, including expectation and Pavlovian conditioning (Benedetti et al., 2005). It is reasonable to assume that the mechanisms by which OLP works are similar to other placebo effects, which likely means activation of brain regions associated with the production and release of hormones and neurotransmitters, leading to physiological changes that can influence exercise performance (Jarcho et al., 2016; Scott et al., 2007). For example, the administration of hidden placebos may influence the release of dopamine, which is, in turn, associated with motivation and willpower (de la Fuente-Fernández et al., 2002) though studies have yet to assess the relevance of increased release of this neurotransmitter in healthy individuals and its impact on sport performance. Furthermore, little is known about whether

OLP causes increased release of catecholamines in a similar way to hidden placebos, but it is plausible to assume that some of the positive effects found in the few studies mentioned above that have assessed the efficacy of OLP on performance outcomes are partly due to this mechanism. Placebo administration may also increase adrenaline and noradrenaline release (Stefano et al., 2001), which influences exercise performance as they alter cardiovascular response (Fredholm et al., 2011), fatty acid mobilisation, glycogen maintenance and perception of pain and perceived exertion (Davis et al., 2003), which combine to improve performance as shown in caffeine studies (Van Soeren et al., 1993). However, mechanistic research is severely lacking, and studies must determine the mechanisms via which OLP works to fully optimise its implementation in a practical setting.

Performance improvements with placebo perceived to be ergogenic substances are well established (Hurst et al., 2020). Placebo pathways appear to act on the same biochemical pathways as the active drug (Finniss et al., 2010), which can be potentialised by expectations and/or conditioning particularly when administered in a therapeutic context. Since OLP does not aim to mimic an active drug, it is difficult to hypothesise plausible mechanisms via which it may act. One aspect through which it may work is by allowing an individual to tap into their physiologic reserve (Corbett et al., 2012; Noakes et al., 2005) via increased motivation and effort. Alternatively, it is possible that the intervention activates certain brain regions involved in the stimulation of neurotransmitters involved in the pathways relevant to exercise performance, such as reward, pain, and pleasure. Likewise, these pathways might directly influence muscle performance. For example, when submitted to an intervention that increases expectation such as a deceptive placebo, an increased release of dopamine can occur (Lidstone et al., 2010), which is a precursor to adrenaline and noradrenaline which can play an important role in muscle contraction. Thus, OLP may work via numerous pathways linked to central and peripheral fatigue, though currently these are speculation and well-controlled mechanistic studies are required to determine the physiological mechanisms that lead to improved performance.

Perspectives

Studies supporting OLP for exercise performance are incipient, but data from clinical research suggest this could be a powerful tool, though confirmatory studies with sport and exercise are required to identify whether this truly is an effective strategy for exercise performance and determine the consistency in response. Several moderating factors may modify the size of the placebo effect (Marticorena et al., 2021). Indeed, preliminary data (Barreto et al., 2021 conference proceedings) suggest that the effect of OLP may be greater in women than in men (effect size, $d = 0.52$ vs. $d = 0.16$, respectively). Determination of the main moderators of this effect are crucial, as well as mechanistic evidence, to optimise this intervention, while screening tools to predict individual responsiveness are desirable. Thus, a directed research program to advance the area is warranted (Saito et al., 2020). The main matters to be resolved include:

1) Whether OLP effectively and consistently elicits ergogenic effects
2) What factors mediate/moderate the effects of this intervention (e.g., sport modalities, training status, sex, physiological characteristics)
3) What mechanisms underpin the effects of OLP
4) What, if any, are the predictors of individuals who respond and those who do not respond

Addressing these gaps will provide more conclusive evidence as to whether OLP can be a useful tool for coaches and athletes to enhance exercise performance in practice.

Conclusions and perspectives

In a sporting context, OLP emerges as an ethically acceptable strategy to improve exercise performance to be used alongside other legal ergogenic aids (e.g., dietary supplements) and/or in replacement of illegal tools (e.g., anabolic steroids). Direct studies on the topic, however, remain limited in number and quality, with methodological differences which preclude current implementation of OLP placebo in the field of sport and exercise.

References

Barreto, G., Saito, T., Oliveira, L. F., Grecco, B., Oliveira, T. N., Merola, P., Carvalho, A., Gualano, B., & Saunders, B. (2021). Apparent sex-differences on the effects of an open-placebo intervention on 4-km time trial performance in trained cyclists. *3rd International Conference of The Society for Interdisciplinary Placebo Studies (SIPS2021) conference*, University of Maryland, Baltimore.

Beedie, C., Benedetti, F., Barbiani, D., Camerone, E., Cohen, E., Coleman, D., Davis, A., Elsworth-Edelsten, C., Flowers, E., & Foad, A. (2018). Consensus statement on placebo effects in sports and exercise: The need for conceptual clarity, methodological rigour, and the elucidation of neurobiological mechanisms. *European Journal of Sport Science, 18*(10), 1383–1389.

Beedie, C. J., & Foad, A. J. (2009). The placebo effect in sports performance: A brief review. *Sports Medicine, 39*, 313–329.

Benedetti, F., Mayberg, H. S., Wager, T. D., Stohler, C. S., & Zubieta, J.-K. (2005). Neurobiological mechanisms of the placebo effect. *Journal of Neuroscience, 25*(45), 10390–10402.

Benedetti, F., Pollo, A., & Colloca, L. (2007). Opioid-mediated placebo responses boost pain endurance and physical performance: Is it doping in sport competitions? *Journal of Neuroscience, 27*(44), 11934–11939.

Canestri, R., Franco-Alvarenga, P. E., Brietzke, C., Vinícius, Í., Smith, S. A., Mauger, A. R., Goethel, M. F., & Pires, F. O. (2021). Effects of experimentally induced muscle pain on endurance performance: A proof-of-concept study assessing neurophysiological and perceptual responses. *Psychophysiology, 58*(6), e13810.

Corbett, J., Barwood, M. J., Ouzounoglou, A., Thelwell, R., & Dicks, M. (2012). Influence of competition on performance and pacing during cycling exercise. *Medicine & Science in Sports & Exercise, 44*(3), 509–515.

Davis, A. J., Hettinga, F., & Beedie, C. (2020). You don't need to administer a placebo to elicit a placebo effect: Social factors trigger neurobiological pathways to enhance sports performance. *European Journal of Sport Science, 20*(3), 302–312.

Davis, J. M., Zhao, Z., Stock, H. S., Mehl, K. A., Buggy, J., & Hand, G. A. (2003). Central nervous system effects of caffeine and adenosine on fatigue. *American Journal of Physiology-Regulatory, Integrative and Comparative Physiology, 284*(2), R399–404.

De Craen, A. J., Roos, P. J., De Vries, A. L., & Kleijnen, J. (1996). Effect of colour of drugs: Systematic review of perceived effect of drugs and of their effectiveness. *BMJ, 313*(7072), 1624–1626.

de la Fuente-Fernández, R., Schulzer, M., & Stoessl, A. J. (2002). The placebo effect in neurological disorders. *The Lancet Neurology, 1*(2), 85–91.

Finniss, D. G., Kaptchuk, T. J., Miller, F., & Benedetti, F. (2010). Biological, clinical, and ethical advances of placebo effects. *The Lancet, 375*(9715), 686–695.

Flowers, K. M., Patton, M. E., Hruschak, V. J., Fields, K. G., Schwartz, E., Zeballos, J., Kang, J. D., Edwards, R. R., Kaptchuk, T. J., & Schreiber, K. L. (2021). Conditioned open-label placebo for opioid reduction after spine surgery: A randomized controlled trial. *Pain, 162*(6), 1828.

Fredholm, B. B., Riksen, N. P., Smits, P., & Rongen, G. A. (2011). The cardiovascular effects of methylxanthines. *Methylxanthines*, 413–437.

Grotle, M., & Hagen, K. B. (2017). Placebo pills provided without deception may help to reduce pain and disability in people with chronic low back pain [synopsis]. *Journal of Physiotherapy, 63*(3), 183.

Guevarra, D. A., Moser, J. S., Wager, T. D., & Kross, E. (2020). Placebos without deception reduce self-report and neural measures of emotional distress. *Nature Communications, 11*(1), 3785.

Hoenemeyer, T. W., Kaptchuk, T. J., Mehta, T. S., & Fontaine, K. R. (2018). Open-label placebo treatment for cancer-related fatigue: A randomized-controlled clinical trial. *Scientific Reports, 8*(1), 2784.

Hurst, P., Schipof-Godart, L., Szabo, A., Raglin, J., Hettinga, F., Roelands, B., Lane, A., Foad, A., Coleman, D., & Beedie, C. (2020). The placebo and nocebo effect on sports performance: A systematic review. *European Journal of Sport Science, 20*(3), 279–292.

Jarcho, J. M., Feier, N. A., Labus, J. S., Naliboff, B., Smith, S. R., Hong, J.-Y., Colloca, L., Tillisch, K., Mandelkern, M. A., & Mayer, E. A. (2016). Placebo analgesia: Self-report measures and preliminary evidence of cortical dopamine release associated with placebo response. *NeuroImage: Clinical, 10*, 107–114.

Kaptchuk, T. J., Friedlander, E., Kelley, J. M., Sanchez, M. N., Kokkotou, E., Singer, J. P., Kowalczykowski, M., Miller, F. G., Kirsch, I., & Lembo, A. J. (2010). Placebos without deception: A randomized controlled trial in irritable bowel syndrome. *PLoS One, 5*(12), e15591.

Kelley, J. M., Kaptchuk, T. J., Cusin, C., Lipkin, S., & Fava, M. (2012). Open-label placebo for major depressive disorder: A pilot randomized controlled trial. *Psychotherapy and Psychosomatics*, *81*(5), 312–314.

Khan, S. I., McNeil, C. J., Gandevia, S. C., & Taylor, J. L. (2011). Effect of experimental muscle pain on maximal voluntary activation of human biceps brachii muscle. *Journal of Applied Physiology*, *111*(3), 743–750.

Lidstone, S. C., Schulzer, M., Dinelle, K., Mak, E., Sossi, V., Ruth, T. J., de la Fuente-Fernández, R., Phillips, A. G., & Stoessl, A. J. (2010). Effects of expectation on placebo-induced dopamine release in Parkinson disease. *Archives of General Psychiatry*, *67*(8), 857–865.

Marticorena, F. M., Carvalho, A., de Oliveira, L. F., Dolan, E., Gualano, B., Swinton, P., & Saunders, B. (2021). Nonplacebo controls to determine the magnitude of ergogenic interventions: A systematic review and meta-analysis. *Medicine and Science in Sports and Exercise*, *53*(8), 1766–1777.

Miller, F. G., & Colloca, L. (2009). The legitimacy of placebo treatments in clinical practice: Evidence and ethics. *The American Journal of Bioethics*, *9*(12), 39–47.

Noakes, T. D., St Clair Gibson, A., & Lambert, E. V. (2005). From catastrophe to complexity: A novel model of integrative central neural regulation of effort and fatigue during exercise in humans: Summary and conclusions. *British Journal of Sports Medicine*, *39*(2), 120–124.

Rossow, L. M., Moon, J., Hiebert, L., Espitia, C., & Fahs, C. A. (2019). The effects of honest and dishonest placebo ingestion immediately prior to VO2peak and handgrip strength testing. *Journal of Trainology*, *8*(2), 27–30.

Saito, T., Barreto, G., Saunders, B., & Gualano, B. (2020). Is open-label placebo a new ergogenic aid? A commentary on existing studies and guidelines for future research. *Sports Medicine*, *50*(7), 1225–1229.

Saunders, B., Saito, T., Klosterhoff, R., de Oliveira, L. F., Barreto, G., Perim, P., Pinto, A. J., Lima, F., de Sá Pinto, A. L., & Gualano, B. (2019). "I put it in my head that the supplement would help me": Open-placebo improves exercise performance in female cyclists. *PLoS One*, *14*(9), e0222982.

Schaefer, M., Harke, R., & Denke, C. (2016). Open-label placebos improve symptoms in allergic rhinitis: A randomized controlled trial. *Psychotherapy and Psychosomatics*, *85*(6), 373–375.

Schaefer, M., Sahin, T., & Berstecher, B. (2018). Why do open-label placebos work? A randomized controlled trial of an open-label placebo induction with and without extended information about the placebo effect in allergic rhinitis. *PLoS One*, *13*(3), e0192758.

Scott, D. J., Stohler, C. S., Egnatuk, C. M., Wang, H., Koeppe, R. A., & Zubieta, J.-K. (2007). Individual differences in reward responding explain placebo-induced expectations and effects. *Neuron*, *55*(2), 325–336.

Stefano, G. B., Fricchione, G. L., Slingsby, B. T., & Benson, H. (2001). The placebo effect and relaxation response: Neural processes and their coupling to constitutive nitric oxide. *Brain Research Reviews*, *35*(1), 1–19.

Swafford, A. P., Kwon, D. P., MacLennan, R. J., Fukuda, D. H., Stout, J. R., & Stock, M. S. (2019). No acute effects of placebo or open-label placebo treatments on strength, voluntary activation, and neuromuscular fatigue. *European Journal of Applied Physiology*, *119*, 2327–2338.

Swinton, P. A., Hemingway, B. S., Saunders, B., Gualano, B., & Dolan, E. (2018). A statistical framework to interpret individual response to intervention: Paving the way for personalized nutrition and exercise prescription. *Frontiers in Nutrition, 5,* 41.

Van Soeren, M., Sathasivam, P., Spriet, L., & Graham, T. (1993). Caffeine metabolism and epinephrine responses during exercise in users and nonusers. *Journal of Applied Physiology, 75*(2), 805–812.

Zhou, E. S., Hall, K. T., Michaud, A. L., Blackmon, J. E., Partridge, A. H., & Recklitis, C. J. (2019). Open-label placebo reduces fatigue in cancer survivors: A randomized trial. *Supportive Care in Cancer, 27,* 2179–2187.

13

IF I INJECT WORDS NOT DRUGS, WILL ATHLETES BE LESS LIKELY TO DOPE?

Philip Hurst and Abby Foad

Introduction

Use of prohibited performance-enhancing substances and methods (i.e., doping), such as anabolic steroids, human growth hormone and blood transfusions, is prevalent across sport (de Hon et al., 2015) and can pose significant health risks (Kanayama et al., 2009; Pope et al., 2014). To circumvent use, the World Anti-Doping Agency (WADA) implements prevention (e.g., anti-doping education), detection (e.g., urine drug testing), and sanction (e.g., excluding athletes from sport) methods to over 200 international and national organisations. In the past decade, WADA has invested over $300 million globally to prevent and deter doping, with a large proportion being used to implement anti-doping education interventions (WADC, 2021). When implemented properly, anti-doping education can provide athletes with information to make more informed decisions about the substances they use. However, while WADA and sport organisations have heavily invested in anti-doping education programmes over the past decade (Woolf, 2020), the effectiveness of current interventions has been questioned (Hoberman, 2013; Hurst et al., 2020b), largely due to a lack of effectiveness in preventing the use of prohibited substances and techniques (Hoberman, 2013; Hurst et al., 2020a; Kavussanu et al., 2021). If WADA is to achieve its aim in preventing doping, effective interventions need to be developed, and employed.

Researchers who study placebo effects in sports performance have argued that evidence for placebo effects can be used as a vehicle to highlight the (lack of) effectiveness of performance-enhancing substances and, in turn, help athletes make a more informed decision prior to use (Beedie & Foad, 2009; Hurst et al., 2017; Hurst et al., 2019b; Hurst et al., 2020b; Kalasountas et al., 2007;

DOI: 10.4324/9781003229001-13

Maganaris et al., 2000; McClung & Collins, 2007). This is on the basis that an athlete may be less likely to consider using a potentially harmful substance after learning that their expectations of, and experience with, a substance or technique can influence how effective it is, irrespective of its innate biological or mechanical properties. In this chapter, we interrogate this idea and examine whether evidence of placebo effects can be used to help guide athletes' decisions towards using prohibited performance-enhancing substances. We will first provide a brief overview of doping in sport and the structures in place aimed at detecting and preventing its use before examining the important role beliefs play in an athlete's decision to dope and how they can influence the effectiveness of a substance. We will then review evidence that suggests athletes may be less likely to dope after either experiencing or even being informed about placebo effects and the influence this has on sport performance. We conclude by proposing methods sport practitioners can adopt to help athletes make more informed decisions about their use of performance enhancing substances.

Doping in sport

The use of substances and methods to improve performance has permeated sport since the beginning of competition. Ancient Olympians (776–394 AD) were reported to have eaten raw animal testicles, hearts, and brains for performance-enhancing purposes (Willick et al., 2016; Yesalis & Bahrke, 2002). In the late 1800s, athletes combined alcohol, strychnine, and heroin to improve performance and drank coffee spiked with cocaine to increase their chances of success (Hoberman, 2001; Yesalis & Bahrke, 2002). While such practices show the significant health risks athletes exposed themselves to, it was only after the amphetamine-related death of Dutch cyclist Knut Jenson in 1960 that the International Olympic Committee published a list of prohibited substances and methods outlining what athletes cannot use (de Hon, 2016).

Up until the end of the twentieth century, most sports organisations would independently implement their own doping policies and sanctions for those athletes failing a drug test. After the 1998 "Festina scandal", in which the Festina cycling team were found to have a systematic doping programme, stakeholders met at the World Conference on Doping in Sport and agreed that an independent organisation is needed to prevent use of prohibited performance-enhancing substances (Dimeo, 2016). As a result, the World Anti-Doping Agency (WADA) was created in 1999, to standardise anti-doping policies across all Olympic sports. Today, while greater resources are allocated to detecting those who are doping than at any previous time, the number of athletes found to have doped has not changed since WADA's inception. Despite the prevalence of doping having been estimated at between 14% and

39% (de Hon et al., 2015), since 1999, the proportion of athletes who fail a drug test has been between 1 and 2% (Gleaves et al., 2021).

Given the above, several researchers have advocated for prevention to take precedence over detection (Backhouse et al., 2018; Kavussanu et al., 2022; Ntoumanis et al., 2014). This is on the basis that preventing a behaviour is more effective than discouraging or punishing one that is already established. Prevention interventions are a cornerstone of WADA's policy (WADC, 2021), and in 2021, the International Standards for Education were published (WADA, 2020). This policy standardises the development and delivery of anti-doping education interventions for stakeholders. Today, anti-doping education is delivered globally across Africa, Asia, Europe, North and South America, and Oceania and a key requirement of the sport organisations involved is to develop and implement effective education interventions that prevent athletes from doping. For anti-doping organisations to develop effective interventions, it is important that they target psychological factors associated with an athlete's decision to dope. In the following section, we highlight the role expectations play in an athlete's decision to use performance-enhancing substances, and how these beliefs can be targeted in anti-doping education interventions.

Expectations, placebo effects and doping

Expectations of performance-enhancing substances are fundamental to various theoretical models of doping (Hauw & McNamee, 2015), with a large body of evidence demonstrating their significant role in an athlete's decision to dope (Backhouse et al., 2016; Ntoumanis et al., 2014).

Hurst et al. (2019a) asked over 1,000 athletes to complete a questionnaire related to performance-enhancing substances and found those who expected performance-enhancing substances to be effective were more likely to use these substances. In fact, researchers found that an athlete may be more likely to use prohibited substances due to the expectation that dietary supplements, which are not prohibited by WADA, improve performance. In a follow-up study, Hurst et al. (2021) found that users of nutritional (e.g., iron) and ergogenic (e.g., caffeine) substances reported more favourable doping attitudes than those who used sport foods and drinks (e.g., electrolytes), and superfoods (e.g., goji berries). Based on this evidence it is therefore reasonable to suggest that substances which have shown greater evidence of effectiveness and, thus, are believed to be more beneficial on sport performance (e.g., caffeine), could lead an athlete to develop more favourable attitudes towards doping than those which have shown little evidence to improve performance (e.g., goji berries).

In the placebo effect literature, expectations have long been associated with the induction of placebo effects (Price et al., 2008). Expectations can often be self-fulfilling; that is, athletes report improvements in performance after using a substance because they expect it will improve performance. A recent systematic review suggests that the strength of placebo effects can depend on how much an athlete expects the purported substance or technique is performance-enhancing (Hurst et al., 2020a). This review suggests that placebo effects about mechanical ergogenic aids (e.g., transcutaneous nerve stimulation) are associated with a larger effect size than placebo effects of purported nutritional ergogenic aids (e.g., caffeine), and that when an athlete has repeated experience of using a substance, placebo effects are larger than when used once, which is suggestive of a conditioning or conditioning-like effect. Placebo effects are smaller for ergogenic aids that have shown little evidence for their effectiveness on sport performance, such as kinesiotape and magnetic wristbands, and are largest for substances prohibited by WADA, such as anabolic steroids and recombinant erythropoietin (EPO). In short, evidence suggests when an athlete uses a performance-enhancing substance, that athlete's expectations of its effectiveness can be a significant factor in the magnitude of any placebo effect.

Collectively, research from both doping and placebo effect literatures highlights the fundamental role expectations play in explaining why a substance is effective and why an athlete may decide to use that substance. For organisations aiming to prevent doping, targeting, and ideally modifying an athlete's expectations via education interventions is likely to have a strong impact on whether that athlete dopes.

Placebo effects as an anti-doping intervention

Much of the early momentum around placebo effect research in sport was the result of debrief interviews with participants, a requirement of the American Psychological Association ethical guidelines on deceptive research (American Psychological Association, 2016). During interview, many participants report that being involved in a study of placebo effects, in which they are administered an inert capsule believing it to be a performance-enhancing substance, changed their beliefs about the mechanisms by which purported performance-enhancing substances might exert their effect (Beedie et al., 2006; Kalasountas et al., 2007; Maganaris et al., 2000). Anecdotal evidence from elite and professional athletes indicate that changes in substance use behaviour might result from experiences with placebos in research (Maganaris et al., 2000) and in real-world competition (Beedie, 2007). Supporting this hypothesis in the substance abuse literature, meta-analytical data indicates that placebo effect interventions can result in reductions of quantity of alcohol consumed and the frequency of heavy drinking (Scott-Sheldon et al., 2012). Fundamentally, this research suggests that placing an athlete in a situation in which they experience a placebo effect of a performance-enhancing substance might modify that athlete's belief in the effectiveness of a substance and in turn, their decision to use it.

Maganaris et al. (2000) were first to highlight that experience of placebo effects could act as a strong deterrent for athletes tempted to use prohibited substances. After deceptively informing national-level weightlifters that they had received an anabolic steroid, authors reported that participants improved the amount of weight lifted in bench press, deadlift, and back squat. Upon being debriefed, participants reported they were less likely to dope and that their desire to use potentially harmful substances, such as anabolic steroids, was curtailed. While this evidence is limited in that it is anecdotal, it highlights the significant influence knowledge of placebo effects can have on athletes' substance use decisions.

Several other researchers have encouraged the importance of using placebo effects as an anti-doping educational tool (Hurst et al., 2020a). After using a balanced placebo design to examine placebo effects on sodium bicarbonate and finding that the belief of using sodium bicarbonate improved performance to the same magnitude as actually taking the substance, McClung and Collins (2007) reported that educating athletes about these results could form the basis of an anti-doping intervention that deters athletes from using prohibited performance-enhancing substances. Similarly, Hurst et al. (2017) reported that athletes who intended to use dietary supplements were more likely to respond to a placebo and encouraged anti-doping organisations to inform athletes that reasons for improvements in performance after using a substance may be the result of their beliefs that they are effective. Likewise, Beedie (2007) reported the testimony of a professional cyclist who had been given a placebo in competition and who had performed above expectation, indicating that the experience had a powerful effect on his attitude towards doping; in short, that the active ingredient had been in his mind and not the capsule.

Given the above, if athletes are informed that placebo effects can affect their performance to a similar degree as performance-enhancing substances, they may be less likely to use these substances in the future and adopt alternative methods in which to achieve their goals. Despite over two decades of researchers suggesting this (Hurst et al., 2020a), no evidence exists of this being implemented in anti-doping education interventions. In the following section, we outline the ways in which this can be achieved and methods that can used in practice to help athletes make more informed choices about their use of performance enhancing substances.

Anti-doping interventions and placebo effects

In this section, we propose two methods practitioners can adopt to help educate athletes about placebo effects. The first outlines how practitioners can embed knowledge and understanding of placebo effects into current anti-doping interventions: the second relates to experiential learning, which can be used in its own right as an anti-doping educational intervention.

Embedding knowledge of placebo effects into anti-doping interventions

Typically, anti-doping education sessions are classroom-based and last between 60 and 90 minutes. Sessions take place in both small and large groups where an anti-doping facilitator provides information about anti-doping including rule violations, drug testing, therapeutic use exemptions, medications, and dietary supplements (Hurst et al., 2020b). In relation to placebo effects, given the majority of research literature has used dietary supplements to highlight its impact on performance, we suggest the facilitator is best placed to embed information about the phenomena at this stage. The facilitator can choose to explain a variety of placebo effect topic areas related to case-studies of athletes reporting placebo effects, its magnitude on sport performance, key mechanisms, and pertinent research findings. We have outlined the ways in which a facilitator can achieve this in Table 13.1 and explain this in more detail below.

TABLE 13.1 Key topics, aims and tasks that facilitators can use to embed into anti-doping interventions

Topic	Aim	Tasks
Introduction to placebo effects	Introduce the placebo effect in relation to performance-enhancing substances	Ask participants what they already know about the placebo effect and if they have ever experienced a placebo effect Provide a layman definition of placebo effects
Real-world examples of placebo effects	Showcase real-life examples of placebo effects in sport	Highlight the examples of Richard Virenque and Willy Voigt Present examples related to athlete beliefs influencing sport performance (e.g., Harry Gallagher, Arsène Wenger) Use videos and stories of athletes exercising a placebo effect
Placebo effect research on sport performance	Describe key findings of placebo effect research	Show the results of research findings (e.g., Maganarais et al., 2000; Beedie et al., 2006; Ross et al., 2015) and systematic reviews (e.g., Hurst et al., 2020b)
	Highlight the magnitude placebo effects have on sport performance	Highlight that the placebo effect can influence performance by, on average, 5.1% Indicate that placebo effects are largest for doping substances
Placebo effects and doping	Question where the effectiveness of doping substances comes from	In groups, ask participants to question the need to use doping substances Present questions as to the benefits of doping substances over and above placebo effects

Once dietary supplements are introduced, the facilitator should indicate that the benefits associated with many supplements such as caffeine, sodium bicarbonate and carbohydrates, can be influenced by placebo effects. At this stage, it is necessary to explain what the placebo effect is and provide a basic definition that a lay audience would understand, such as "an improvement in performance because of the belief that a dietary supplement is beneficial". To highlight its significance in sport, the facilitator should provide real-world examples of athletes having experienced a placebo effect and the impact this has had on their performance. The most notable example includes the cyclist Richard Virenque being injected with glucose believing it to be a performance-enhancing substances, and stating that it significantly improved his performance (Voet, 2001). Other examples have been reported elsewhere related to Olympic swimming coach, Harry Gallagher, doctoring the stopwatches so that his athletes believed they were performing to a higher level and the football coach, Arsène Wenger, injecting his players with benign vitamins that they believed significantly improved their performance (Merson & Allen, 2011). To confirm understanding, the facilitator should ask the audience what they know about the placebo effect and if they believe they have ever experienced it.

Once the placebo effect has been introduced, the facilitator should highlight key placebo effect research. To ensure the audience can fully understand the results, it is suggested the facilitator uses examples that are relatively straightforward to understand, and the message is not overly complicated. Such example includes Maganaris et al. (2000), who reported that national-level weightlifters increased the amount of weight they could lift by 4.6% and improved to an international level after taking a placebo believed to be an anabolic steroid and Ross et al., (2015), who reported that athletes ran 1.5% quicker when they injected saline that they believed was a recombinant erythropoietin-like substance. Afterwards, the facilitator can present the results of a systematic review to highlight placebo effects can improve performance (Hurst et al., 2020a). At this point it would be worthwhile for the facilitator to indicate that placebo effects are likely to have a larger influence on banned performance-enhancing substances, such as anabolic steroids and erythropoietin, compared to dietary supplements, including caffeine and sodium bicarbonate. The facilitator should conclude the session by asking the group to discuss the significant role placebo effects can have on the effectiveness of performance-enhancing substances. Such discussion questions to consider are: Why do placebo effects appear to be larger for prohibited substances, such as anabolic steroids, than permitted substances, such as caffeine? If placebo effects have been shown to improve performance up to 5%, are performance-enhancing substances needed? Instead of using a prohibited performance-enhancing substance, what could an athlete do to improve performance?

While we have provided an outline of how information about placebo effects can be embedded into anti-doping interventions, facilitators can be flexible in choosing what topics to include in their sessions (Table 13.1); provided that the audience is informed about the influence placebo effects can have on the effectiveness of performance-enhancing substances. To help convey information and maximise engagement with the content, where possible, facilitators are encouraged to use real-life stories relating to placebo effects and provide examples specific to the audience's sport.

Placebo effects and experiential learning

Arguably, an athlete, upon learning about placebo effects and their role in the effectiveness of a performance-enhancing substance, is likely to question where the effectiveness of that substance comes from and conclude that such substances may not be needed to meet their goals. Thus, many researchers have suggested that experiencing a placebo effect, and learning about it, could be used as a strong anti-doping education intervention (Hurst et al., 2020a). This type of education is based on experiential learning, which recognises the importance of the self as a source of information (Kolb, 1984). A placebo effect experiential learning intervention would therefore involve an athlete participating in a placebo effect experiment and, upon being debriefed about the true nature of that experiment, reflecting on their experiences during it.

Implementing an experiential learning intervention in practice presents significant challenges. By nature, placebo effect research requires asking athletes to standardise their lifestyle over the course of an experiment (e.g., diet, sleep, training), provide consistent information to each participant about the study, and multiple site visits. Placebo effects are also frequently examined within complex designs, such as the balanced placebo design (Foad et al., 2008; Hurst et al., 2019) and conditioning paradigms (Benedetti & Dogue, 2015; Benedetti et al., 2007; Pollo et al., 2008). Implementing this in practice would be resource-intensive, require expert knowledge and take time away from an athlete's regimented training programme. As a result, experiential educational interventions need to be simple, specific to the requirements of an athlete's sport and completed in a timeframe that does not interrupt intense training schedules and practices.

Unlike most placebo effect research, Beedie et al. (2007) used a pre-post-test design to directly induce placebo effects in a large sample of athletes on repeated sprint performance. Authors asked athletes to run 3 × 30-m sprints with a short recovery, before randomising them to two belief groups: 1) positive and 2) negative. They then administered placebos to the athletes and informed the positive belief group that it would improve performance and the negative belief group that it would worsen performance. Twenty minutes later, athletes ran another 3 × 30-m sprints and results showed that those in the positive belief group ran progressively faster over the final three sprints, whereas those in the negative belief group ran progressively slower.

This study highlights a simple but effective method in which to induce placebo effects in a sample of athletes within a short timeframe (~30 minutes). Results can be received instantly through timing gates or stopwatches, involves repeated sprinting that is inherent in most sports (e.g., football, Rugby union, cricket) or training programmes and has implications for how athletes understand the impact placebo effects can have on speed, power, and fatigue.

The experiential learning intervention would commence once the athlete completes the repeated sprints and is debriefed about the true nature of it. This would take shape in three distinct phases. First, once the deception has been revealed, the results of the trial should be shown to athletes upon which they are then asked to reflect on their own performance and consider why their performance may have changed. Second, athletes are then asked to consider similar situations where placebo effects may have occurred (e.g., through using medications, dietary supplements or other training apparel and equipment) and critically reflect on whether performance improvements were a result of using that method or placebo effects. Finally, athletes are asked to consider the need to use performance enhancing substances when benefits may be the result of placebo effects and identify other ways in which performance can be improved via, for example, psychological strategies, training methods, nutrition, or sleep.

Summary

At its core, placebo effect research is related to how beliefs about an intervention (e.g., anabolic steroids improve performance) can influence the effectiveness of that intervention. While some have warned placebo effect research can be problematic for the sport and exercise community (Beedie et al., 2018: see also Beedie's chapter in this book) in the context of anti-doping, evidence of placebo effects can be a powerful tool in highlighting the significant influence an athlete's belief can have in the effectiveness of performance-enhancing substances. Empirical evidence from both placebo effect and anti-doping literature has highlighted that an athlete is likely to use a performance-enhancing substance and respond positively to it because of the belief it improves performance. This highlights an important mechanism to target for those interested in preventing doping in sport.

In this chapter we have outlined ways in which organisations can use knowledge and understanding of placebo effects to help athletes make more informed decisions about the use of performance-enhancing substances. We have highlighted ways in which anti-doping practitioners can complement and strengthen existing interventions by giving athletes the opportunity to *learn* about and *experience* the placebo effect. Together, educational and experiential approaches can help shape an athlete's belief about the effectiveness of performance-enhancing substances and enable them to make better, more informed decisions about the use of these substances.

References

American Psychological Association. (2016). Ethical principles of psychologists and code of conduct. *American Psychologist, 57*(12), 1060–1073.

Backhouse, S., Whitaker, L., Patterson, L., Erickson, K., & McKenna, J. (2016). Social Psychology of Doping in Sport: A Mixed Studies Narrative Synthesis. Project Report. World Anti-Doping Agency, Montreal Canada.

Backhouse, S. H., Griffiths, C., & McKenna, J. (2018). Tackling doping in sport: a call to take action on the dopogenic environment. *British Journal of Sports Medicine, 52,* 1485–1486. https://doi.org/10.1136/bjsports-2016-097169

Beedie, C. (2007). Placebo effects in competitive sport: Qualitative data. *Journal of Sports Science & Medicine, 6*(1), 21.

Beedie, C. J., Coleman, D. A., & Foad, A. J. (2007). Positive and negative placebo effects resulting from the deceptive administration of an ergogenic aid. *International Journal of Sport Nutrition and Exercise Metabolism, 17*(3), 259–269.

Beedie, C. J., & Foad, A. J. (2009). The placebo effect in sports performance: A brief review. *Sports Medicine, 39,* 313–329.

Beedie, C. J., Stuart, E. M., Coleman, D. A., & Foad, A. J. (2006). Placebo effects of caffeine on cycling performance. *Medicine and Science in Sports and Exercise, 38*(12), 2159.

Benedetti, F., & Dogue, S. (2015). Different placebos, different mechanisms, different outcomes: Lessons for clinical trials. *PLoS One, 10*(11), e0140967.

Benedetti, F., Pollo, A., & Colloca, L. (2007). Opioid-mediated placebo responses boost pain endurance and physical performance: Is it doping in sport competitions? *Journal of Neuroscience, 27*(44), 11934–11939.

de Hon, O. (2016). *Striking the right balance.* Utrecht University.

de Hon, O., Kuipers, H., & van Bottenburg, M. (2015). Prevalence of doping use in elite sports: A review of numbers and methods. *Sports Medicine, 45*(1), 57–69. https://doi.org/10.1007/s40279-014-0247-x

Dimeo, P. (2016). The myth of clean sport and its unintended consequences. *Performance Enhancement & Health, 4*(3–4), 103–110. https://doi.org/10.1016/j.peh.2016.04.001

Foad, A. J., Beedie, C. J., & Coleman, D. A. (2008). Pharmacological and psychological effects of caffeine ingestion in 40-km cycling performance. *Medicine and Science in Sports and Exercise, 40*(1), 158.

Gleaves, J., Petróczi, A., Folkerts, D., De Hon, O., Macedo, E., Saugy, M., & Cruyff, M. (2021). Doping prevalence in competitive sport: Evidence synthesis with "best practice" recommendations and reporting guidelines from the WADA working group on doping prevalence. *Sports Medicine, 51*(9), 1909–1934.

Hauw, D., & McNamee, M. (2015). A critical analysis of three psychological research programs of doping behaviour. *Psychology of Sport and Exercise, 16,* 140–148. https://doi.org/10.1016/j.psychsport.2014.03.010

Hoberman, J. (2013). How much do we (really) know about anti-doping education? *Performance Enhancement & Health, 2*(4), 137–143. https://doi.org/10.1016/j.peh.2014.09.002

Hoberman, J. M. (2001). *Mortal engines: The science of performance and the dehumanization of sport.* Blackburn Press.

Hurst, P., Foad, A., Coleman, D., & Beedie, C. (2017). Athletes intending to use sports supplements are more likely to respond to a placebo. *Medicine & Science in Sports & Exercise (MSSE), 49*(9), 1877–1888.

Hurst, P., Kavussanu, M., Boardley, I., & Ring, C. (2019a). Sport supplement use predicts doping attitudes and likelihood via sport supplement beliefs. *Journal of Sports Sciences, 37*(15), 1734–1740. https://www.embase.com/search/results? subaction=viewrecord&id=L628365467&from=export

Hurst, P., Ring, C., & Kavussanu, M. (2020a). Evaluation of UK athletics clean sport programme in preventing doping in junior elite athletes. *Performance Enhancement & Health, 7*(4), 1–6. https://doi.org/10.1016/j.peh.2019.100155

Hurst, P., Ring, C., & Kavussanu, M. (2021). Athletes using ergogenic and medical sport supplements report more favourable attitudes to doping than non-users. *Journal of Science and Medicine in Sport, 24*(3), 307–311. https://doi.org/10. 1016/j.jsams.2020.09.012

Hurst, P., Schipof-Godart, L., Hettinga, F., Roelands, B., & Beedie, C. (2019b). Improved 1000-m running performance and pacing strategy with caffeine and placebo: A balanced placebo design study. *International Journal of Sports Physiology and Performance, 15*(4), 483–488.

Hurst, P., Schipof-Godart, L., Szabo, A., Raglin, J., Hettinga, F., Roelands, B., Lane, A., Foad, A., Coleman, D., & Beedie, C. (2020b). The placebo and nocebo effect on sports performance: A systematic review. *European Journal of Sport Science, 20*(3), 279–292.

Kalasountas, V., Reed, J., & Fitzpatrick, J. (2007). The effect of placebo-induced changes in expectancies on maximal force production in college students. *Journal of Applied Sport Psychology, 19*(1), 116–124.

Kanayama, G., Brower, K. J., Wood, R. I., Hudson, J. I., & Pope, H. G., Jr. (2009). Anabolic-androgenic steroid dependence: An emerging disorder. *Addiction, 104*(12), 1966–1978. https://doi.org/10.1111/j.1360-0443.2009.02734.x

Kavussanu, M., Barkoukis, V., Hurst, P., Yukhymenko, M., Skoufa, L., Chirico, A., Lucidi, F., & Ring, C. (2022). A Psychological intervention reduces doping likelihood in british and greek athletes: A Cluster randomized controlled trial. *Psychology of Sport & Exercise, 61*, 102099.

Kavussanu, M., Hurst, P., Yukhymenko-Lescroart, M., Galanis, E., King, A., Hatzigeorgiadis, A., & Ring, C. (2021). A moral intervention reduces doping likelihood in UK and greek athletes: Evidence from a cluster randomized control trial. *Journal of Sport & Exercise Psychology, 43*(2), 125–139. https://doi.org/10.1123/ jsep.2019-0313

Kolb, D. A. (1984). *Experiential learning: Experience as the source of learning and development.* Prentice Hall.

Maganaris, C. N., Collins, D., & Sharp, M. (2000). Expectancy effects and strength training: Do steroids make a difference? *The Sport Psychologist, 14*(3), 272–278.

McClung, M., & Collins, D. (2007). "Because I know it will!": Placebo effects of an ergogenic aid on athletic performance. *Journal of Sport and Exercise Psychology, 29*(3), 382–394.

Merson, P., & Allen, M. (2011). *How not to be a professional footballer.* HarperSport London.

Ntoumanis, N., Ng, J. Y., Barkoukis, V., & Backhouse, S. (2014). Personal and psychosocial predictors of doping use in physical activity settings: A meta-analysis. *Sports Medicine, 44*(11), 1603–1624. https://doi.org/10.1007/s40279-014-0240-4

Pollo, A., Carlino, E., & Benedetti, F. (2008). The top-down influence of ergogenic placebos on muscle work and fatigue. *European Journal of Neuroscience, 28*(2), 379–388.

Pope, H. G., Jr., Wood, R. I., Rogol, A., Nyberg, F., Bowers, L., & Bhasin, S. (2014). Adverse health consequences of performance-enhancing drugs: An Endocrine Society scientific statement. *Endocrine Reviews*, *35*(3), 341–375. https://doi.org/10.1210/er.2013-1058

Price, D. D., Finniss, D. G., & Benedetti, F. (2008). A comprehensive review of the placebo effect: Recent advances and current thought. *Annual Review of Psychology*, *59*, 565–590. https://doi.org/10.1146/annurev.psych.59.113006.095941

Ross, R., Gray, C. M., & Gill, J. M. (2015). The effects of an injected placebo on endurance running performance. *Medicine and Science in Sports and Exercise*, *47*(8), 1672–1681.

Scott-Sheldon, L. A., Terry, D. L., Carey, K. B., Garey, L., & Carey, M. P. (2012). Efficacy of expectancy challenge interventions to reduce college student drinking: A meta-analytic review. *Psychology of Addictive Behaviors*, *26*(3), 393–405. https://doi.org/10.1037/a0027565

Voet, W. (2001). Breaking the chain. *Drugs and Cycling–The True Story, Yellow*.

WADA. (2020). 2021 International Standard for Education.

WADC. (2021). The world anti-doping code. https://www.wada-ama.org/sites/default/files/resources/files/wada-2015-world-anti-doping-code.pdf

Willick, S. E., Miller, G. D., & Eichner, D. (2016). The Anti-Doping Movement. *PMR*, *8*(3 Suppl), S125–S132. https://doi.org/10.1016/j.pmrj.2015.12.001

Woolf, J. J. R. (2020). An examination of anti-doping education initiatives from an educational perspective: Insights and recommendations for improved educational design. *Performance Enhancement & Health*, 100178.

Yesalis, C. E., & Bahrke, M. S. (2002). History of doping in sport. *International Sports Studies*, *24*(1), 42–76.

14

IS IT OK TO RECOMMEND COMPLEMENTARY OR ALTERNATIVE MEDICINE EVEN THOUGH I KNOW IT'S A PLACEBO?*

Why the neurobiology of the placebo effect does not legitimise the use of CAM

Chris Beedie

Introduction

Evidence-based medicine (EBM) is arguably the cornerstone of medicine and sports medicine. Acceptable sources of evidence include the peer-reviewed scientific literature, in which findings of clinical trials and research studies are often reported in relation to a placebo control treatment, and in which patient case studies and similar are vetted by experts (Djulbegovic & Guyatt, 2017). Historically, many 'traditional' treatments, consisting of, or based on, naturally occurring substances, have been subjected to randomised controlled trials. Many have performed better than placebo controls and are therefore today classified as medicine. Treatments that have either not yet been subjected to randomised controlled trials (RCTs) – or which have been subjected to RCTs and have not consistently performed better than a placebo – are often termed 'complimentary and/or alternative medicines' (CAM). The term 'complementary medicine' suggests use alongside evidence-based medicine (also termed 'integrative' treatment), whilst the term 'alternative medicine' suggests use instead of EBM. Not surprisingly, CAM is a broad category with examples including homeopathy, magnetic mattresses, and acupuncture.

Complementary and alternative medicine

Use of CAM is currently widespread across the world (Tangkiatkumjai et al., 2020). Data from the 2017 National Health Interview Survey found that

---

* An abbreviated version of this chapter has been published previously in the British Journal of Sports Medicine (Beedie et al., 2017), which has been approved by the publisher.

DOI: 10.4324/9781003229001-14

prevalence of CAM increased in the past decade from 9.5% to 14.3% (Clarke et al., 2018), with rates in populations such as cancer patients even higher, reported between 43% and 87% (Judson et al., 2017; Sanford et al., 2019). When used alongside conventional treatments, potential benefits of CAM include a greater sense of treatment benefit and improved quality of life (Rhee & Harris, 2018), the reduction and/or management of drug side effects (Hershman et al., 2018), and the reduced risk of dependence on drugs such as opioids (Kroenke & Cheville, 2017). The downsides of CAM include:

1. The risk of harm from untested treatments, even those described as 'natural'.
2. Interactions when used alongside conventional therapies (West, 2018).
3. The likelihood that people receiving CAM might decline conventional treatments even in potentially fatal illness such as cancer (Johnson et al., 2018).
4. The risk of developing a reliance on what is to all intents a ritual or token.

Evidence for the effectiveness of various CAM treatments has been published in many discrete studies. However, systematic reviews highlight serious methodological limitations common to many, for example the absence of placebo controls, small sample sizes, poor experimental design and high risk of bias (Bardia et al., 2006; Close et al., 2014; Hohenauer et al., 2015; Hussain & Quigley, 2006; Lee et al., 2008; Mostafavifar et al., 2012) (Long et al., 2020; Mathie et al., 2014). Of reviews that report what the authors describe as reliable findings, many support the idea that specific CAM treatments are entirely a placebo (Friesen, 2019), for example homeopathy (Shang et al., 2005), are ineffective, for example electromagnetic therapy (McCarthy et al., 2006), or that data are uninterpretable, for example chiropractic procedures (Lesho, 1999).

Complimentary alternative medicine in sport

Although evidence for CAM is highly contentious, prevalence among athletes is often reported as one of the highest among various user groups (Koh et al., 2012). Of a survey of 257 sports medicine physicians (Kent et al., 2020), 88% reported prescribing at least one type of CAM in the previous year. Respondents identified 23 different type of CAM prescription, including chiropractic/osteopathic manipulation, acupuncture & electroacupuncture, yoga, omega-3 fatty acids, riboflavin, and meditation. These were prescribed for what the authors described as common sports medicine pathologies, including ligamentous, tendinous and muscle injury, concussion, and low back pain, among others. The authors concluded that many survey participants believed many of these CAM modalities to be effective. In another survey of 334 athletes

(Rotter et al., 2021), 69% reported use of at least one type of CAM within the last 12 months, with osteopathy, herbal medicine, vitamins/minerals, and relaxation techniques the most frequently used. A notable example of the use of CAM in sport is provided by Michael Phelps, the USA swimmer who at the time of writing in 2023 remains the most successful Olympic athlete in history with 23 Olympic gold medals. Phelps' evident use of cupping at the 2016 Olympic Games (Musumeci, 2016) drew widespread media attention. While cupping, which is the use of heated glass bowls intended to improve blood circulation, is likely relatively harmless – although harm has been reported (Seifman et al., 2017) – other CAM widely used in sport, such as natural and synthetic ergogenic aids, can be potentially harmful, as can medicines and/or procedures developed for clinical applications that are used without evidence of efficacy or safety in sport.

The evidence for CAM in sport mirrors that in medicine, whereby there is a significant lack of robust evidence to support its effectiveness. Some evidence for the benefits of CAM include, for example, kinesio taping (Lim & Tay, 2015) and cold-water immersion (Machado et al., 2016), but methodological problems within these studies are commonplace, such as the lack of appropriate blinding (Bailey et al., 2009; Fratocchi et al., 2013; Rowsell et al., 2014). Similarly, many well-controlled studies of CAM suggest no benefits beyond placebo, for example acupuncture (Urroz et al., 2016), cold-water immersion (Broatch et al., 2014), hologram wristbands (Brazier et al., 2014), ischemic preconditioning (Marocolo et al., 2016), kinesio taping (Poon et al., 2015), normobaric hypoxia (Siebenmann et al., 2011), respiratory muscle training (Sonetti et al., 2001), and ultrasound (Ulus et al., 2012).

To satisfactorily address issues relating to CAM in sport, it would be impossible to address the full range of CAM treatments within the scope of this chapter. Instead, the focus of the discussion is directed to the example of dietary supplements (e.g., caffeine, protein drinks, vitamins and minerals), which are widely used by athletes of all ages and abilities (Knapik et al., 2016). This is despite the fact that the dietary supplement industry is largely unregulated and rarely provides any evidence for the effectiveness or safety of their products (Maughan, 2013). Products are attractive to the consumer as they are legally available and often marketed as 'natural', 'organic' or 'pure', and athletes may therefore assume that they are safe and effective. Contrary to this, however, such products can contain substances associated with documented health risks. For example, a review of 24 commercially available protein drinks indicated that 31% failed quality assurance tests, with 6 to 18 mg of lead discovered in some of the products (Maughan, 2013). Likewise another study reported that products sold online did not include any of the active ingredients displayed on the label, with low-cost and potentially dangerous substitutes such as melamine used instead of protein ingredients (Champagne & Emmel, 2011). The use of a weight-loss CAM containing hidden quantities of an untested drug (n-nitroso-fenfluramine) resulted in four deaths and 800 people falling seriously ill (McVeigh et al., 2012; Zell-Kanter et al., 2015), and a similar weight-loss supplement (ephedra) has been linked to multiple deaths and cardiovascular incidences (Zell-Kanter et al., 2015). It has been suggested that the contamination of such products is not necessarily the result of poor quality control, but might equally be the result of deliberate adulteration of products to enhance their efficacy (Maughan, 2005).

Given the above, the Australian Institute of Sport's (AIS) Supplement Framework (https://www.ais.gov.au/nutrition/supplements) has proposed four classifications:

- Group A: Approved supplements that have shown strong scientific evidence for their effectiveness and safety and include, for example, bicarbonate, caffeine, and carbohydrate drinks.
- Group B: Supplements under consideration that require further research before they can be confidently classified as beneficial and safe for use by athletes, including fruit derived polyphenols, menthol and ketones.
- Group C: Supplements with no clear proof of beneficial effects and are not advocated for use by athletes, which include the majority of other substances promoted to athletes and non-athletes alike, such as branch chain amino acids (BCAA), B-Hydroxy B-Methylbutyrate (HMB) and magnesium.
- Group D: Substances prohibited by the World Anti-Doping Agency, which include ephedrine, androgenic anabolic steroids and beta-2-agonists.

Why mechanisms for the placebo effect are not per se mechanisms of CAM

With the emergence of research into placebo effects in the last two decades, consistent neurobiological mechanisms have been reported (Beedie et al., 2020; see also chapter by Roelands in this book). Alongside this, emerging data has highlighted interesting trends and methodological innovations relating to the study of placebo effects showing that the effects in the placebo arm of clinical trials are increasing in number year on year (Tuttle et al., 2015). Perhaps more counterintuitively, the open-label administration of placebos – presenting the placebo with full disclosure to the patient that the treatment they are about to receive is a placebo – is likewise associated with positive effects on health and sport performance outcomes (see chapter by Saunders in this book). Several plausible hypotheses might explain both, but one that cannot be ignored is the increasing sense among everyday people, and therefore among participants in clinical trials, that placebos are somehow powerful in their own right (Tuttle et al., 2015), that, whether they have been consigned to the placebo arm of the trial, or even openly administered a placebo, participants expect a positive effect.

The results of both medical and sport research on placebos have, in some senses at least, legitimised placebo effects, shifting its status from vague and contested psychosocial phenomenon controlled for in RCTs, to a cluster of predictable and measurable neurobiological events. However, given the strong connection between placebo effects and CAM, the idea that the growing mechanistic evidence for placebo effects de facto signifies growing mechanistic evidence for CAM has gained traction among practitioners and the media.[1] This idea has also been articulated, albeit in not quite such explicit terms, in the medical literature (Kaptchuk, 2002; Kaptchuk & Miller, 2005). Whilst many practitioners would dismiss the idea that CAM is legitimised via placebo effects, others would suggest, as does Kaptchuk (Kaptchuk, 2002; Kaptchuk & Miller, 2005), that if CAM results in an improvement, then a treatment effect has been observed, even more so if a physiological or neurobiological mechanism for that improvement can be identified.

And herein lies the crux of the issue. The placebo effect is now associated with clear neurobiological mechanisms. It could be argued, therefore, that practitioners of any treatment which relies upon placebo effects could cite those mechanisms as evidence for the efficacy of the treatment itself. Whilst at face value this is not entirely illegitimate, and while we do not wish to discount the potential of placebo effects to inform future practice or constitute treatments in their own right, I contest this position, and propose five challenges to the idea that placebo mechanisms legitimise the use of CAM by athletes:

1. Variability in placebo responsiveness: Arguably, when a treatment with a legitimate biological effect is administered to a placebo-responsive individual it is augmented by the placebo effect, and when administered to a non-placebo responsive individual, the only effect is the biological effect of the treatment. However, in the case of a CAM treatment, by definition, any biological effect is likely absent. While the treatment might still result in a positive effect on a placebo responsive patient, there will be no effect if administered to a patient who is not placebo-responsive, or who has no expectations of, or prior conditioning experience with, the treatment in question. A treatment reliant on placebo effects, if administered to a non-responsive individual is, de facto, no treatment. But is there such a thing as a placebo-responsive athlete? Placebo responding is variable, both between and within individuals (Beedie et al., 2008). Some individuals might be more likely to respond to a placebo than others, but this might vary between situations such as pre-match to treatment table, between practitioners, for example strength and conditioning coach and physiotherapist, and between contexts, for example performance enhancement and injury rehabilitation. Variability in response to deceptive treatments has been previously reported in sport (Beedie et al., 2008; Hurst et al., 2017; Seligman et al., 1990).

Furthermore, most research examines the placebo effect in acute contexts, and little is known about the stability of placebo effects in sport over time. This might not be a critical factor in a unique one-off scenario, for example the use of a CAM treatment to deal with, for example, acute pain, but is important in many, if not most sports medicine contexts where treatment is extended over time. In short, although a placebo effect might exert a significant influence on a performance or an individual treatment, there is little evidence that it will continue to do so.

2. Potential for placebos to have a negative effect: It has been suggested that if a placebo treatment was submitted to a drug agency for approval, although the agency would be impressed with the efficacy data, it would probably be disapproved on the basis of the high incidence of side effects (Glasser & Frishman, 2008). Data indicate that nocebo effects, that is a negative outcome related to negative expectations or experience, is as much a possibility in many situations as a positive placebo effect (see chapter by Colloca in this book). In short, practitioners, far from being confident that using a treatment will invariably result in an improvement in performance, must consider the possibility that administration of a placebo treatment can exert a negative effect. Pre-existing beliefs about, or experiences with, a certain treatment can result in negative effects of a substance that entirely eliminate therapeutic benefits. In 2006, for example, a participant in a study of the placebo effects of caffeine in cycling performance discontinued the study due to his having experienced nausea and headache as the result of the high level of caffeine he believed he had received (Beedie et al., 2006). He had been administered a placebo presented as likely to have a positive effect on his performance, but his expectations based on previous experience with caffeine likely played a role in his experiencing a nocebo effect. Such expectations and experiences are rarely factored into either research or practice. More importantly, the assumption that because a treatment is presented as positive and/or beneficial does not mean that the athlete will see it the same way (ask any dentist). Although the intentions of practitioners may be benevolent, this benevolence may not always result in a positive outcome.

3. Ethics relating to not recommending/adopting a more effective treatment. Perhaps the most frequently cited objection to the use of CAM in medical practice is that patients who choose CAM might at the same time choose to not use more effective and/or evidence-based treatments (Smith et al., 2016). In sport, this might range from an athlete not eating sufficient fresh fruit on the basis that they are ingesting sufficient vitamin C through supplements, often referred to as a "licensing effect", to choosing CAM as opposed to conventional medicine to treat serious injury or illness. It has been recognised that sports medicine practitioners do not have a strong evidence base for some of what they do (Orchard et al., 2008), and also

that "elite athletes are a vulnerable group often happy to accept at face value a treatment purported to expedite their return to play for a variety of factors" (Franklyn-Miller et al., 2011). Therefore, encouraging reliance among athletes on treatments that may prevent them seeking more appropriate and potentially more effective nutritional, lifestyle, training, psychological or even medical approaches presents ethical concerns.

4. Ethics of deception: Even if the above are ignored, there remain significant ethical problems with the deliberate administration of a placebo intervention (see chapter by Campos, Borry and McNamee (chapter 15)). These issues go beyond those related to evidence-based practice and the lack of evidence for many CAM treatments, and are addressed in depth elsewhere (Benedetti, 2012; Finniss et al., 2010; Miller et al., 2004). To knowingly advocate CAM while at the same time knowing that the only likely mechanism of effect is the placebo, is unethical, even if only for the reasons given in points 1 and 2 above. Whilst arguments as to the ethics of the deliberate deception of clients by professionals, even in a good cause, are beyond the scope of this chapter, to do so would certainly breach many professional practice guidelines. I acknowledge that there are some data which have found open-label administration of placebos to be effective in medicine (Kaptchuk et al., 2010), but these results are presently limited to a small range of clinical conditions (e.g., Irritable Bowel Syndrome) and in sports performance (see chapter by Bryan Saunders). In short, whilst it is ethically problematic to deceive, it is perhaps less ethically problematic to state for example, "This is a complementary treatment, if it works, it is likely because of a placebo effect", or alternatively "This is a placebo, placebos have been found to enhance the performance of athletes in previous research by around 3%". But these are speculative. This is an issue for future ethical debate, but should also be considered in the light of points 1 and 2 above, and of the last point below, that whilst it might be ethical, it might still be ultimately counterproductive.

5. Identification of alternative "headroom" mechanisms: Lastly, a critical question surrounding the capacity of any individual to respond to a placebo should be this: the capacity to respond to a placebo, manifest as an improvement in performance or performance-related variable, is evidence of headroom between current and potential performance. The headroom in question is arguably the result of one or more deficits or inefficiencies in performance physiology or psychology, which are likely amenable to a legitimate treatment, be that physiological (e.g., training, recovery, skill/technique, nutrition) or psychological (e.g., self-belief, arousal regulation, self-awareness, pain tolerance). It should be the goal of the athlete and/or practitioner to seek to identify and capitalise on such headroom through legitimate, controllable, and stable methods such as optimal nutrition, systematic training and recovery, and emotional/psychological skills training.

Summary

The mechanism underlying many CAM treatments is arguably a result of placebo effects. Although most forms of CAM are not prohibited in sport, their use poses pragmatic and ethical questions. At the core of the issue is the question of what constitutes a legitimate treatment. Many have argued for the potential of the placebo effect in medicine and in sport (Beedie et al., 2015; Roelands & Hurst, 2020). We have no doubt that there will soon be sufficient understanding of the multivariate components of placebo responsiveness to allow evidence-based practitioners to use placebo pathways transparently and ethically in enhancing health and/or performance. At such a time, some CAM might become legitimate components of medicine. However, such advances in treatment would require substantial empirical evidence, as well as revisions to ethical and professional guidelines for practice. Until that time we maintain that CAM can be effective but it can also be harmful, that evidence is vague in both respects, and that practitioners and athletes using CAM do not always recognise this.

Placebo effects that underlie many CAM treatments are unstable and unpredictable, varying in magnitude and direction both between and within individuals. While we acknowledge the argument that, in sports performance, the effect – even if only a placebo – is often more important than the mechanism, we caution that in using many forms of CAM, even a placebo effect is not assured, a direct biological treatment effect even less so. On this basis, in using CAM, an athlete might simply be wasting resources – financial, time, energy, emotional – unnecessarily, be placing their health and performance at risk, either as the result of direct factors such as contamination, or indirectly because they may use CAM as a substitute for healthy behaviours, and, through their reliance on external and unstable treatments, might fail to develop internal and stable psychological and/or physiological capacities to bring about the desired outcome.

With robust evidence, CAM is no longer CAM, it is re-classified as evidence-based medicine. The type of evidence necessary for this to occur may include new understanding of the neurophysiology of placebo effects. Sports medicine researchers and practitioners should seek to use robust, reliable, and, where necessary, innovative methods to evaluate the efficacy and mechanisms of CAM treatments used in sport and should not rely on non-specific effects as a basis for prescription. Non-evidence-based treatments should be used with caution and in light of the five warnings above. It might be going too far to suggest that such treatments should be labelled with the statement "Caution: This treatment is a placebo, it may not work for a number of reasons, and might even be counter-productive", but we argue this is most certainly the reality that practitioners should keep in mind if doing so.

Note

1 I have been researching the placebo effect in sport for 20 years. Whilst it is not unusual to be invited to speak at scientific conferences or to the media about one's area of expertise, I receive as many invitations to speak on the issue of CAM, and an equal volume of emails and social media traffic from proponents and/or practitioners of CAM, at times congratulating me for legitimising and/or promoting their product or treatment.

References

Bailey, S. J., Winyard, P., Vanhatalo, A., Blackwell, J. R., Dimenna, F. J., Wilkerson, D. P., Tarr, J., Benjamin, N., & Jones, A. M. (2009). Dietary nitrate supplementation reduces the O2 cost of low-intensity exercise and enhances tolerance to high-intensity exercise in humans. *Journal of Applied Physiology (1985)*, *107*(4), 1144–1155. https://doi.org/10.1152/japplphysiol.00722.2009

Bardia, A., Barton, D. L., Prokop, L. J., Bauer, B. A., & Moynihan, T. J. (2006). Efficacy of complementary and alternative medicine therapies in relieving cancer pain: A systematic review. *Journal of Clinical Oncology*, *24*(34), 5457–5464. https://doi.org/10.1200/JCO.2006.08.3725

Beedie, C., Benedetti, F., Barbiani, D., Camerone, E., Lindheimer, J., & Roelands, B. (2020). Incorporating methods and findings from neuroscience to better understand placebo and nocebo effects in sport. *European Journal of Sport Science*, *20*(3), 313–325.

Beedie, C., Foad, A., & Hurst, P. (2015). Capitalizing on the Placebo Component of Treatments. *Current Sports Medicine Reports*, *14*(4), 284–287. https://doi.org/10.1249/JSR.0000000000000172

Beedie, C., Whyte, G., Lane, A.M., Cohen, E., Raglin, J., Hurst, P., Coleman, D., & Foad, A. (2018). 'Caution, this treatment is a placebo. It might work, but it might not': why emerging mechanistic evidence for placebo effects does not legitimise complementary and alternative medicines in sport. *British Journal of Sports Medicine*, *52*(13), 817–818.

Beedie, C. J., Foad, A. J., & Coleman, D. A. (2008). Identification of placebo responsive participants in 40km laboratory cycling performance. *Journal of Sports Science and Medicine*, *7*(1), 166–175. http://www.ncbi.nlm.nih.gov/pubmed/24150150

Beedie, C. J., Stuart, E. M., Coleman, D. A., & Foad, A. J. (2006). Placebo effects of caffeine on cycling performance. *Medicine and Science in Sports and Exercise*, *38*(12), 2159.

Benedetti, F. (2012). The placebo response: Science versus ethics and the vulnerability of the patient. *World Psychiatry*, *11*(2), 70–72. http://www.ncbi.nlm.nih.gov/pubmed/22654931

Brazier, J., Sinclair, J., & Bottoms, L. (2014). The effects of hologram wristbands and placebo on athletic performance *Kinesiology 46*(1), 109–116.

Broatch, J. R., Petersen, A., & Bishop, D. J. (2014). Postexercise cold water immersion benefits are not greater than the placebo effect. *Medicine & Science in Sports & Exercise*, *46*(11), 2139–2147.

Champagne, A. B., & Emmel, K. V. (2011). Rapid screening test for adulteration in raw materials of dietary supplements. *Vibrational Spectroscopy*, *55*(2), 216–223. https://doi.org/10.1016/j.vibspec.2010.11.009

Clarke, T. C., Barnes, P. M., Black, L. I., Stussman, B. J., & Nahin, R. L. (2018). *Use of yoga, meditation, and chiropractors among US adults aged 18 and over.* US Department of Health and Human Services, Centers for Disease Control and ....

Close, C., Sinclair, M., Liddle, S., Madden, E., McCullough, J., & Hughes, C. (2014). A systematic review investigating the effectiveness of Complementary and Alternative Medicine (CAM) for the management of low back and/or pelvic pain (LBPP) in pregnancy. *Journal of Advanced Nursing, 70*(8), 1702–1716.

Djulbegovic, B., & Guyatt, G. H. (2017). Progress in evidence-based medicine: A quarter century on. *The Lancet, 390*(10092), 415–423. https://doi.org/10.1016/S0140-6736(16)31592-6

Finniss, D. G., Kaptchuk, T. J., Miller, F., & Benedetti, F. (2010). Biological, clinical, and ethical advances of placebo effects. *Lancet, 375*(9715), 686–695. https://doi.org/10.1016/S0140-6736(09)61706-2

Franklyn-Miller, A., Etherington, J., & McCrory, P. (2011). Sports and exercise medicine--specialists or snake oil salesmen? *British Journal of Sports Medicine, 45*(2), 83–84. https://doi.org/10.1136/bjsm.2009.068999

Fratocchi, G., Di Mattia, F., Rossi, R., Mangone, M., Santilli, V., & Paoloni, M. (2013). Influence of Kinesio Taping applied over biceps brachii on isokinetic elbow peak torque. A placebo controlled study in a population of young healthy subjects. *Journal of Science and Medicine in Sport, 16*(3), 245–249. https://doi.org/10.1016/j.jsams.2012.06.003

Friesen, P. (2019). Mesmer, the placebo effect, and the efficacy paradox: Lessons for evidence based medicine and complementary and alternative medicine. *Critical Public Health, 29*(4), 435–447.

Glasser, S. P., & Frishman, W. (2008). The placebo and nocebo effect. In S. P. Glasser (Ed.), *Essentials of clinical research* (pp. 111–140). Springer Netherlands. https://doi.org/10.1007/978-1-4020-8486-7_7

Hershman, D. L., Unger, J. M., Greenlee, H., & et al. (2018). Effect of acupuncture vs sham acupuncture or waitlist control on joint pain related to aromatase inhibitors among women with early-stage breast cancer: A randomized clinical trial. *JAMA, 320*(2), 167–176. https://doi.org/10.1001/jama.2018.8907

Hohenauer, E., Taeymans, J., Baeyens, J. P., Clarys, P., & Clijsen, R. (2015). The Effect of Post-Exercise Cryotherapy on Recovery Characteristics: A Systematic Review and Meta-Analysis. *PLos One, 10*(9), e0139028. https://doi.org/10.1371/journal.ponc.0139028

Hurst, P., Foad, A. J., Coleman, D., & Beedie, C. (2017). Athletes intending to use sports supplements are more likely to respond to a placebo. *Medicine & Science in Sports & Exercise, 49*(9), 1877–1883.

Hussain, Z., & Quigley, E. M. (2006). Systematic review: Complementary and alternative medicine in the irritable bowel syndrome. *Alimentary Pharmacology & Therapeutics, 23*(4), 465–471. https://doi.org/10.1111/j.1365-2036.2006.02776.x

Johnson, S. B., Park, H. S., Gross, C. P., & Yu, J. B. (2018). Complementary medicine, refusal of conventional cancer therapy, and survival among patients with curable cancers. *JAMA Oncology, 4*(10), 1375–1381. https://doi.org/10.1001/jamaoncol.2018.2487

Judson, P. L., Abdallah, R., Xiong, Y., Ebbert, J., & Lancaster, J. M. (2017). Complementary and alternative medicine use in individuals presenting for care at a comprehensive cancer center. *Integrative Cancer Therapies, 16*(1), 96–103.

Kaptchuk, T. J. (2002). The placebo effect in alternative medicine: Can the performance of a healing ritual have clinical significance? *Annals of Internal Medicine 136*(11), 817–825. https://doi.org/10.7326/0003-4819-136-11-200206040-00011

Kaptchuk, T. J., Friedlander, E., Kelley, J. M., Sanchez, M. N., Kokkotou, E., Singer, J. P., Kowalczykowski, M., Miller, F. G., Kirsch, I., & Lembo, A. J. (2010). Placebos without deception: A randomized controlled trial in irritable bowel syndrome. *PLoS One, 5*(12), e15591. https://doi.org/10.1371/journal.pone.0015591

Kaptchuk, T. J., & Miller, F. G. (2005). Viewpoint: What is the best and most ethical model for the relationship between mainstream and alternative medicine: Opposition, integration, or pluralism? *Academic Medicine, 80*(3), 286–290. https://doi.org/10.1097/00001888-200503000-00015

Kent, J., Tanabe, K. O., Muthusubramanian, A., Statuta, S. M., & MacKnight, J. M. (2020). Complementary and Alternative Medicine Prescribing Practices Among Sports Medicine Providers. (1078–6791 (Print)).

Knapik, J. J., Steelman, R. A., Hoedebecke, S. S., Austin, K. G., Farina, E. K., & Lieberman, H. R. (2016). Prevalence of Dietary Supplement Use by Athletes: Systematic Review and Meta-Analysis. *Sports Medicine, 46*(1), 103–123. https://doi.org/10.1007/s40279-015-0387-7

Koh, B., Freeman, L., & Zaslawski, C. (2012). Alternative medicine and doping in sports. *The Australasian Medical Journal, 5*(1), 18–25. https://doi.org/10.4066/AMJ.20121079

Kroenke, K., & Cheville, A. (2017). Management of chronic pain in the aftermath of the opioid backlash. *JAMA, 317*(23), 2365–2366. https://doi.org/10.1001/jama.2017.4884

Lee, M. S., Pittler, M. H., & Ernst, E. (2008). Effects of reiki in clinical practice: A systematic review of randomised clinical trials. *International Journal of Clinical Practice, 62*(6), 947–954. https://doi.org/10.1111/j.1742-1241.2008.01729.x

Lesho, E. P. (1999). An overview of osteopathic medicine. *Archives of Family Medicine, 8*(6), 477–484. https://doi.org/10.1001/archfami.8.6.477

Lim, E. C., & Tay, M. G. (2015). Kinesio taping in musculoskeletal pain and disability that lasts for more than 4 weeks: Is it time to peel off the tape and throw it out with the sweat? A systematic review with meta-analysis focused on pain and also methods of tape application. *British Journal of Sports Medicine, 49*(24), 1558–1566.

Long, Y., Chen, R., Guo, Q., Luo, S., Huang, J., & Du, L. (2020). Do acupuncture trials have lower risk of bias over the last five decades? A methodological study of 4 715 randomized controlled trials. *PLoS One, 15*(6), e0234491.

Machado, A. F., Ferreira, P. H., Micheletti, J. K., de Almeida, A. C., Lemes, I. R., Vanderlei, F. M., Netto Junior, J., & Pastre, C. M. (2016). Can Water Temperature and Immersion Time Influence the Effect of Cold Water Immersion on Muscle Soreness? A Systematic Review and Meta-Analysis. *Sports Medicine, 46*(4), 503–514. https://doi.org/10.1007/s40279-015-0431-7

Marocolo, M., Willardson, J. M., Marocolo, I. C., Ribeiro da Mota, G., Simao, R., & Maior, A. S. (2016). Ischemic Preconditioning and Placebo Intervention Improves Resistance Exercise Performance. *The Journal of Strength and Conditioning Research, 30*(5), 1462–1469. https://doi.org/10.1519/JSC.0000000000001232

Musumeci, G. (2016). Could cupping therapy be used to improve sports performance? *Journal of Functional Morphology and Kinesiology, 1*(4), 373–377.

Mathie, R. T., Lloyd, S. M., Legg, L. A., Clausen, J., Moss, S., Davidson, J. R., & Ford, I. (2014). Randomised placebo-controlled trials of individualised homeopathic treatment: Systematic review and meta-analysis. *Systematic Reviews*, *3*, 1–16.

Maughan, R. J. (2005). Contamination of dietary supplements and positive drug tests in sport. *Journal of Sports Sciences*, *23*(9), 883–889. https://doi.org/10.1080/02640410400023258

Maughan, R. J. (2013). Quality assurance issues in the use of dietary supplements, with special reference to protein supplements. *Journal of Nutrition*, *143*(11), 1843S–1847S.

McCarthy, C. J., Callaghan, M. J., & Oldham, J. A. (2006). Pulsed electromagnetic energy treatment offers no clinical benefit in reducing the pain of knee osteoarthritis: A systematic review. *BMC Musculoskelet Disord*, *7*(1), 51. https://doi.org/10.1186/1471-2474-7-51

McVeigh, J., Evans-Brown, M., & Bellis, M. A. (2012). Human enhancement drugs and the pursuit of perfection. *Adicciones*, *24*(3), 185–190. http://www.ncbi.nlm.nih.gov/pubmed/22868973

Miller, F. G., Emanuel, E. J., Rosenstein, D. L., & Straus, S. E. (2004). Ethical issues concerning research in complementary and alternative medicine. *JAMA*, *291*(5), 599–604. https://doi.org/10.1001/jama.291.5.599

Mostafavifar, M., Wertz, J., & Borchers, J. (2012). A systematic review of the effectiveness of kinesio taping for musculoskeletal injury. *Phys Sportsmed*, *40*(4), 33–40. https://doi.org/10.3810/psm.2012.11.1986

Orchard, J. W., Best, T. M., Mueller-Wohlfahrt, H. W., Hunter, G., Hamilton, B. H., Webborn, N., Jaques, R., Kenneally, D., Budgett, R., Phillips, N., Becker, C., & Glasgow, P. (2008). The early management of muscle strains in the elite athlete: Best practice in a world with a limited evidence basis. *British Journal of Sports Medicine*, *42*(3), 158–159. https://doi.org/10.1136/bjsm.2008.046722

Poon, K. Y., Li, S. M., Roper, M. G., Wong, M. K., Wong, O., & Cheung, R. T. (2015). Kinesiology tape does not facilitate muscle performance: A deceptive controlled trial. *Manual Therapy*, *20*(1), 130–133.

Rhee, T. G., & Harris, I. M. (2018). Reasons for and perceived benefits of utilizing complementary and alternative medicine in U.S. adults with migraines/severe headaches. *Complementary Therapies in Clinical Practice*, *30*, 44–49. https://doi.org/10.1016/j.ctcp.2017.12.003

Roelands, B., & Hurst, P. (2020). The placebo effect in sport: How practitioners can inject words to improve performance. *International Journal of Sports Physiology and Performance*, *15*(6), 765–766.

Rotter, G., Schollbach, L., Binting, S., Dornquast, C., Scherr, J., Pfab, F., & Brinkhaus, B. (2021). Use of complementary medicine in competitive sports: Results of a cross-sectional study. *Complementary Medicine Research*, *28*(2), 139–145. https://doi.org/10.1159/000511247

Rowsell, G. J., Reaburn, P., Toone, R., Smith, M., & Coutts, A. J. (2014). Effect of run training and cold-water immersion on subsequent cycle training quality in high-performance triathletes. *The Journal of Strength and Conditioning Research*, *28*(6), 1664–1672. https://doi.org/10.1519/JSC.0000000000000455

Sanford, N. N., Sher, D. J., Ahn, C., Aizer, A. A., & Mahal, B. A. (2019). Prevalence and nondisclosure of complementary and alternative medicine use in patients with cancer and cancer survivors in the United States. *JAMA Oncology*, *5*(5), 735–737.

Seifman, M. A., Alexander, K. S., Lo, C. H., & Cleland, H. (2017). Cupping: The risk of burns. *Medical Journal of Australia, 206*(11), 500. https://doi.org/10.5694/mja17.00230

Seligman, M. E. P., Nolen-Hoeksema, S., Thornton, N., & Thornton, K. M. (1990). Explanatory Style as a Mechanism of Disappointing Athletic Performance. *Psychological Science, 1*(2), 143–146. http://pss.sagepub.com/content/1/2/143.abstractN2

Shang, A., Huwiler-Muntener, K., Nartey, L., Juni, P., Dorig, S., Sterne, J. A., Pewsner, D., & Egger, M. (2005). Are the clinical effects of homoeopathy placebo effects? Comparative study of placebo-controlled trials of homoeopathy and allopathy. *Lancet, 366*(9487), 726–732. https://doi.org/10.1016/S0140-6736(05)67177-2

Siebenmann, C., Robach, P., Jacobs, R., Rasmussen, P., Nordsborg, N., Diaz, V., Christ, A., Olsen, N., Maggiorini, M., & Lundby, C. (2011). Live high-train low using normobaric hypoxia: A double-blinded, placebo-controlled study. *Journal of Applied Physiology, 112*(1), 106–117.

Smith, K., Ernst, E., Colquhoun, D., & Sampson, W. (2016). 'Complementary & Alternative Medicine' (CAM): Ethical And Policy Issues. *Bioethics, 30*(2), 60–62. https://doi.org/10.1111/bioe.12243

Sonetti, D. A., Wetter, T. J., Pegelow, D. F., & Dempsey, J. A. (2001). Effects of respiratory muscle training versus placebo on endurance exercise performance. *Respiration Physiology, 127*(2–3), 185–199. http://www.ncbi.nlm.nih.gov/pubmed/11504589

Tangkiatkumjai, M., Boardman, H., & Walker, D.-M. (2020). Potential factors that influence usage of complementary and alternative medicine worldwide: A systematic review. *BMC Complementary Medicine and Therapies, 20*(1), 1–15.

Tuttle, A. H., Tohyama, S., Ramsay, T., Kimmelman, J., Schweinhardt, P., Bennett, G. J., & Mogil, J. S. (2015). Increasing placebo responses over time in U.S. clinical trials of neuropathic pain. *Pain, 156*(12), 2616–2626. https://doi.org/10.1097/j.pain.0000000000000333

Ulus, Y., Tander, B., Akyol, Y., Durmus, D., Buyukakincak, O., Gul, U., Canturk, F., Bilgici, A., & Kuru, O. (2012). Therapeutic ultrasound versus sham ultrasound for the management of patients with knee osteoarthritis: A randomized double-blind controlled clinical study. *International Journal of Rheumatic Diseases, 15*(2), 197–206. https://doi.org/10.1111/j.1756-185X.2012.01709.x

Urroz, P., Colagiuri, B., Smith, C. A., Yeung, A., & Cheema, B. S. (2016). Effect of acupuncture and instruction on physiological recovery from maximal exercise: A balanced-placebo controlled trial. *BMC Complementary and Alternative Medicine, 16*, 227. https://doi.org/10.1186/s12906-016-1213-y

West, H. (2018). Complementary and alternative medicine in cancer care. *JAMA Oncology, 4*(1), 139–139. https://doi.org/10.1001/jamaoncol.2017.3120

Zell-Kanter, M., Quigley, M. A., & Leikin, J. B. (2015). Reduction in ephedra poisonings after FDA ban. *The New England Journal of Medicine, 372*(22), 2172–2174. https://doi.org/10.1056/NEJMc1502505

15

CAN I USE THE PLACEBO EFFECT TO TREAT INJURED OR ILL ATHLETES?

Ethics, deception, and placebo effects in sports medicine

Marcus Campos, Pascal Borry, and Mike McNamee

Introduction

Placebo studies have recently become an interdisciplinary research topic in sports science and sports medicine, arising from an intensification of scientific findings of placebo mechanisms during the first decade of this century. Beyond medical science, humanistic analysis is essential to assess the desirability of new treatments. This chapter focuses on the ethics of using deceptive placebos in clinical practice (broadly conceived of as sports healthcare practices). These practices are conducted by sports physicians and sports nutritionists, physiotherapists, or other relevantly applicable specialisation. In this chapter, we develop four related themes. First, we analyse the traditional definitions of the placebo effect and its consequences for ethical analysis. Secondly, we showcase what sports medicine entails and why we should bring together evidence to understand it separately from medicine in general. Thirdly, we present the general principles of medical ethics and bioethics and apply them to sports medicine. Fourthly, we close with an understanding of the ethical problems surrounding the use of placebos in sports. We conclude by showing new avenues of investigation that suggest how placebo effects can come in different formats that defy the deceptive paradigm, presenting ethical alternatives for using placebos in clinical practice.

The traditional definition(s) of placebo effects

We begin with some remarks on how placebo effects are understood in relation to medicine or healthcare practice more generally. Traditional definitions of placebo effects often include two necessary conditions. First, placebo effects are understood to be biologically "inert/innocuous". This element is understood

DOI: 10.4324/9781003229001-15

alongside the effects being understood as a form of "treatment".[1] This enables their being, or potentially being aligned with that widespread goal of medicine. In this vein, Brody (2018, p. 354) defines placebos as a "bodily change due to the symbolic effects of a treatment or treatment situation and not to its pharmacologic or physiologic properties". Although a universally agreed definition of treatment is difficult to attain, it is commonly agreed that medicine's goal is the relief of suffering (Porter, 2004). By extension, a definition of treatment refers to an intervention that has as its goal to relieve suffering. Placebo administrations are often coherent with such a goal.

The majority of the placebo literature defines the placebo effect by pairing it with the notion of treatment. Yet the placebo effect has also been defined in a negative way (Alfano, 2015) because of its inert/innocuous aspect. In philosophy, a negative definition is one that employs the opposition or absence of a term as its necessary condition. This method is evidenced in some placebo definitions. For example, for Guijarro (2015, p. 68) a "placebo is a treatment designed to simulate a medical intervention, but which does not exert a biological effect on the disease in question". Whereas, Grünbaum's (1981) widely accepted conception of placebo effects as inert, has the consequence that placebo effects are those not identified by the dominant therapeutic theory. Nocebo effects can also include negative definitions in relation to its inert/innocuous aspect. Yet they are also negative in relation to treatment, since they are expectations derived from a "procedure intended to create negative expectations (e.g., giving a placebo along with verbal suggestions of worsening)" (Miller & Colloca, 2011, p. 598).

More recently, scholars and scientists have drawn attention to a putative characteristic of the received understanding of placebo effects, noting that an alternative understanding arises when we focus on the notion of placebo responses. The intensification of scientific findings related to placebo effects, and the establishment of neurobiological pathways associated with them, has raised questions of which side effects are to be thought of as placebo effects and which are associated with other variables present in the clinical encounter, such as regression to mean, patients' natural history, or bias. In what follows we accept this differentiation and follow Evers' line of reasoning:

> (…) the *placebo and nocebo response* includes all health changes (i.e., differences in symptoms before and after treatment), thus including natural history and regression to the mean. The *placebo and nocebo effect*[, therefore,] refers to the changes specifically attributable to placebo and nocebo mechanisms, including the neurobiological and psychological mechanisms of expectancies.
>
> *(Evers et al., 2018, p. 206)*

As we will show, these aspects of the traditional definitions of placebo effects conflict with and present issues for the ethical assessment of its use in clinical practice. While deemed "inert/innocuous", a placebo can be considered "a substance provided to a patient that the physician believes has no specific pharmacological effect upon the condition being treated" (Bostick et al., 2008, p. 3). Therefore, their administration, usually combined with or in replacement of treatment, is considered deceptive and conflicts with patients' right to information through the informed consent process (Miller & Colloca, 2011). Moreover, because they are parasitic upon the more fundamental "treatment", it is unclear to which extent placebos may be ethically administered, such as the performance enhancement of elite athletes. Thus, it is questionable to what extent, and under which conditions, the use of placebo is ethically acceptable, for example the relief or management of pain, and whether their ethical use extends beyond treatment. An important question therefore exists in relation to what would justify their use for non-medical needs?

One possibility is to point to emerging empirical evidence that challenges the received "inert/innocuous" condition and holds that the placebo effects are genuine neurobiological mechanisms (Colloca, 2014). In that case, some may argue that this opens the door to their ethical use in performance enhancement (Carlino et al., 2014).

Understanding the problems with the use of (deceptive) placebos in clinical practice

Imagine the following scenario related to pain management in a clinical setting. A sports club physician administers a pill to an athlete after complaints of muscular pain after a hard training session. The physician chooses his words carefully to emphasise the positive aspect he wants her to grasp from his evaluation of a specific pill he appears to intend to prescribe: "This is a strong analgesic that has been extremely effective in cases such as yours." Not long after ingestion, the athlete reports positive effects in that she is feeling relief from her pain and more confident about the day's training session. Although the physician intervened with the athlete's best interests at heart, since experience and recent evidence on placebo effects suggest that sham administrations have a great potential to relieve pain, the situation represents a classic example of paternalistic intervention – where the athlete is deceived, but in the name of a beneficent cause – the relief of negatively perceived pain. How are we to evaluate this intervention by the physician. We can ask: (a) is apparent treatment one that sport physicians are apt to conduct; and (b) is it ethically justified? As to the former question, McNamee et al. (2017) argue that it appears part of the professional arsenal of physicians. They cite a highly experienced surgeon working in sports medicine:

> That's where the art of medicine comes in [...] we have patients with overload injuries or they are over-trained, maybe, and you'd like to take them out for three months and that's a lifetime for them. Then, you have to put

on something that you do to avert their attention and to get them to do something other than their usual use […] I think this goes on in every aspect of medicine, I think because there are so many things that we think we know but we don't' know […] Any clinician will use placebo as part of their medication, so to speak. Any experienced physician.

(2017, p. 357)

What of the question as to its ethical status? Deception is often included as a component of the placebo administration. Now here our clinician has skated a thin line; the physician has certainly directed the understanding of the athlete patient in a way that has undermined their autonomy. Moreover, it is commonly held that such deception or – at least – misdirection, is an important aspect in the modulation of the expectation that evoked the response, its administration is ethically problematic. This is because the right to information, the right of patient autonomy, their capacity to form a conception of their own best interests and express these to their healthcare providers, should generate a duty of respect in the healthcare provider (Beauchamp & Childress, 2019). The usurpation of that right may be conceived of as an ethical violation, or in some jurisdictions a legal one. Finally, although the patient responded successfully to the intervention, she *could* have presented negative side effects, namely, nocebo effects. Accordingly, these interrelated issues represent a variety of challenges that the literature on medical ethics have tried to respond to over recent years. They may be summarised into the following topics of investigation: prevalence and physicians' attitudes towards placebos, patients' right to consent, codes and policies in medical care in sports, and the consistency of the evidence on placebo effects in the scientific literature (Kaptchuk et al., 2020).

Together, these issues exemplify some of the potential moral conflicts for clinical practice. However, the most central and discussed issue regarding the use of placebos in clinical practice is deception, defined as "to intentionally cause to have a false belief that is known or believed to be false" (Mahon, 2016). While inadvertently or mistakenly deceiving others would not describe the physicians' example, intention in deceiving is a central problem for clinical practice's legitimacy. Particularly, intentionally deceiving patients can infringe on their right to information and consent (Beauchamp & Childress, 2019). Therefore, it is pressing to understand sports medicine clinical practice and arguments underpinning the moral status of the use of placebos.

Pain, performance, and athletes

Placebo research is often related to pain and less frequently to performance enhancement (Colloca & Benedetti, 2005). In sports, pain and enhancement are an everyday preoccupation for sports healthcare professionals (SHP), where there is highly subjective preference prioritisation. However, most research on placebo effects in sports is related to performance enhancement (Beedie & Foad, 2009; Hurst et al., 2020). Greater attention to the ethical use of placebos for pain management is therefore warranted. We shall assume what is a commonplace in western medical practice that where treatment is concerned, the patients' right to informed consent is paramount. The extension of that principal technique, to assisting performance enhancement, is a moot point.

The IOC Consensus Statement on pain management defines pain as "An unpleasant sensory and emotional experience associated with actual or potential tissue damage, or described in terms of such damage" (Raja et al., 2020). Pain can be either acute or chronic. The presence of chronic pain often renders the athlete a contender for retirement. Athletes reports of life playing with pain are legion. Nor are they restricted to the obvious contenders in collision and contact sports (Nixon, 1992; Huizenga, 1995). Take, for example, Rafael Nadal's statement after being defeated by Denis Shapovalov at the ATP Masters 1000 Rome of 2022: "I am a player living with an injury; it is nothing new." Living with pain and playing in a condition that is not pain-free are part and parcel of everyday elite sports (Howe, 2003). Even though pain is ineliminable from the human condition and a physical mechanism to protect individuals, elite athletes are more exposed to both acute and chronic pain than the average population.

In contact and collision sports, pain is entirely foreseeable.[2] While some see value in the so-called "dangerous sports", others question the moral justifications of some of them, such as boxing or MMA, since their "goal (…) is to win by incapacitating opponents so that they are unable to fight back" (Russell, 2005). Whichever ethical stance is adopted on the intentional infliction of injury and therefore pain on one's opponent, there is no denying its ubiquitous presence. And, of course, it may be self-inflicted in sports that are essentially parallel tests. It is close to received wisdom in endurance cycling (e.g., the European tours) that the winner is often the cyclist who can endure the greatest pain, and therefore inflict the greatest suffering on their opponent.

Regardless of their moral status, all previous examples illustrate how pain is somewhat permissible within the realm of sports. Pain is a central preoccupation of sports medicine due to the prevalence in which athletes are exposed to risks of injury. Pain management is one of the essential components of the care of elite athletes. Conceived broadly, this has implications also for recuperative and preventative practices and not merely therapeutic management (Hainline et al., 2017).

What is surprising, however, is the lacuna of research on using placebos for pain in sports, especially in the light of clinical discussion and when compared to other, non-sport, medical specialisations. Beyond sports, there is widespread use of placebos for pain management. For example, surveys in Denmark (over 80%) and the US (over 50%) have demonstrated that a large number of physicians from different specialisations, such as general practitioners, hospital clinicians, private specialists, or rheumatologists, respond positively when asked of the administration of placebos in the previous year (Hróbjartsson & Norup, 2003).

A preoccupation in sports medicine is the enhancement of performance. Unlike pain management, ethical consideration of performance enhancement often derives from its use as a form of cheating. Much of the available litera-ture is related to the use of performance-enhancing drugs (PEDs) and their corrupt administration among sports participants (Murray, 2015). Concerning placebos, research in sports has shown how nutritional ergogenic aids might enhance performance by evoking the neurobiological mechanisms related to the placebo effects (see chapter by Roelands in this book). More important for our purposes are the evidence of its use for enhancing performance. Adminis-tration of placebos in sports medical settings is common. For example, Brooling et al. (2008) found that 62% of a sample of 30 national-level coaches have allegedly administered placebos to their athletes at some point, while 10% of them proceeded with weekly administrations. This evidence is reinforced by Szabo and Müller's (2016) study, in which 90% of a sample of 96 coaches were aware of placebo effects, while 44% admitted administering placebos to their athletes in an attempt (successful or otherwise) to enhance their performance. However, these administrations need to be considered apart since coaches do not always or easily fit the SHPs category. Moreover, only some authors have addressed the issue from a moral point of view in understanding the relation-ship between placebos and doping (Kayser, 2020; Kirkwood, 2014).

The medical setting in sports and its particular aspects

Whether placebos are a problem for sports medicine (and for sports) requires understanding if there is any difference between them and general medical practice. Sports medicine has been considered to possess some peculiar aspects concerning athletes' health (Malcolm, 2005). This status can be represented by the link some have made between sports medicine physicians as "snake oil salesmen" (Franklyn-Miller et al., 2011). While medicine's goal has been widely conceived as the relief of suffering, this prominent precondition seems to be inconsistent with the variety of activities carried out by physicians (Edwards & McNamee, 2006), since sports medicine practitioners often oper-ate in the grey zones between treatment and performance enhancement (Morgan, 2009).

Although sports medicine is a recent newcomer to the family of medical specialisms, some might argue that it differs from many traditional branches in terms of its conceptual and practical goals. In 2006, Steven D. Edwards and Mike McNamee challenged the class inclusion claim that sports medicine is a branch of medicine. The authors made a point by arguing that for a practice to fall within the class of medicine, "it is necessary that it possess the attribute of aiming to relieve suffering" (Edwards & McNamee, 2006). Conceptually speaking, to be considered a medicine, sports medicine shall attend to the necessary condition of the class: the relief of suffering. While sports medicine is usually conceived as a 'branch of medicine' and a discipline concerned with athletes' welfare and health through prevention, protection, and correction of injuries, as the *Oxford Dictionary of Sports Science & Medicine* states, among its objectives, it includes the practice of preparing "an individual for physical activity in its full range of intensity" or the study of information "used to optimize performance in sports" (Kent, 2006, p. 521).

Capturing daily activities of sports medicine also conflicts with the claim that sports medicine is medicine. Although public discourse often shares the social image of the athletes' body as "health" – e.g., in sports such as swimming or track and field where "fitness" is often understood (incorrectly) as synonymous with "health" – this standardised conception of athletes' body does not show all of the functions an SHP exercises within elite sports contexts. For example, in football, SHP are not only concerned with athletes' recovery from injuries (often sport-related) or illnesses (usually non-sport-related), but with the numerous training sessions, and given the tight championship calendars, highly compressed recovery timeframes. Moreover, the permissiveness of the "machine-like" conception of the athletes' bodies (Gleyse, 2013) also offers conflicts with the elusive assumption that sports medicine coheres uniformly with the goals of medicine.

Sport medicine is not infrequently considered a practice at the borders of medicine. Two characteristics of sport illustrate this borderline status, both commonplace scenarios faced by SHPs. First, from a legal point of view, athletes' mindset to enhance performance and their willingness to put their health at risk by consenting to participate in dangerous practices is an essential factor in the complexity of the everyday life of sports clinical contexts. In sports such as Rugby or skiing, athletes accept the gratuitous logical structure underpinning the contest (Suits, 2014); that is to say, they undertake tasks that are made more complex by the nature and rules of the activity. In some cases, this means that they consent to the legitimisation of risk of serious harm inflicted upon them (Parry, 1998; Dixon, 2016). Due to the risk of many athletes lives coexist with (often extreme) pain while trying to maintain or enhance performance. Secondly, from a sociological standpoint, athletes' willingness to live with pain is part of the culture of risk associated with the sport (Nixon, 1992), represented by what has been called "sportsnets", the social structure surrounding the clinical context of sport in which coexistence with pain is maintained. While such culture has been investigated through numerous normative lenses, such as confidentiality in sports settings (Waddington et al., 2019), less has been said about specific procedures, such as the use of placebos by SHPs.

The, albeit ambiguous, distinction between treatment and enhancement (Buchanan, 2011; Parens, 1995) might give some a platform to argue that sports medicine is unique but still within the family of medical specialisms, yet this claim is flawed. In fact, claims of distinctness or uniqueness are exaggerated (McNamee & Morgan, 2015): "what really exist are merely differences of degree, not differences of kind" (Camporesi & McNamee, 2017, p. 745). Therefore, sports medicine and other branches of medicine are ethically assessed by the same principles, and physicians should comply with the same medical principles. The question then arises as to how we ethically evaluate placebos within sport medicine thus conceived.

Ethical principles for medicine and sports medicine

To guide decision-making when ethical dilemmas appear in medical practice, mainstream medical ethics and bioethics have drawn heavily on principles as opposed to case-by-case casuistic processes. Tools for practical guidance help us to assess complex cases to comprehend SHPs' obligations, limits, or justifications, as well as the rationale behind healthcare policies in sports. Since the 1970s, medical ethics and bioethics literature have relied extensively on principle-based approach (Ainslie, 2002). It was with the publication of *Principles of Biomedical Ethics*, in 1979, that Tom L. Beauchamp and James Childress "not only played a pivotal part in creating the field but for the past 40 years (…) have remained two of its most influential figures" (Shea, 2020). Their four-principles approach to bioethics, also called "principlism", is the most influential approach in the fields of western medical ethics and bioethics, entailing appropriate correspondence to fields such as medicine and sports medicine. Moreover, Beauchamp and Childress' focus on what they call mid-level principles have served as pivotal guides in understanding the ethical issues related to placebo effects, from RCT (Annoni, 2018) to clinical practice (Annoni & Miller, 2016; Miller & Colloca, 2011).

The four principles articulated by Beauchamp & Childress (2019) to guide clinical practice are (i) respect for autonomy, (ii) non-maleficence, (iii) beneficence, and (iv) justice. All four derived from what the authors have called the common morality's approach. In reality, they draw from different moral philosophical sources. While respect for persons and non-maleficence draw from deontological (duty-based) ethics, aiming to benefit the patient (typically expressed at the best interests of the patient) is a guide as to consequential considerations, albeit based on a duty-like formulation. The focus on justice is often a critical issue in the allocation of scarce resources, allowing for a rational basis concerning who gets what in terms of healthcare. Let us elaborate a little further before moving to application specifically concerning placebo use.

The use of placebos by SHPs potentially breaches the widely accepted principles of respect for autonomy (patients' right to choose the treatment) and beneficence (physician's duty to act in the patients' best interest). Autonomy occupies a central place in contemporary moral and political philosophical theories, especially in discussions such as the principles of justice, the limits of free speech, or the nature of liberal states (Dworkin, 2017). Notwithstanding this, the concept of autonomy has been regarded as a pivotal element in practical and applied ethics, such as medical ethics and bioethics, especially in discussions about decision-making and informed consent (Beauchamp & Childress, 2019). According to Beauchamp and Childress (2019), virtually all theories of autonomy support two essential conditions: liberty and agency (the possibility of rational choice over, and responsibility for, one's actions). While the former represents independence from external control, the latter represents the capacity to decide what actions to do intentionally independently.

While the principle of non-maleficence owes its roots to the Hippocratic Oath of the early Greek physicians and was canonised in the classical period with the latin motto *"primum non-nocere"* (first do no harm), it is important to understand that the role of this principle is understood both as a goal and a constraint on physician's action. By contrast, beneficence has to do with undertaking beneficial actions or promoting good. It was, in previous decades, a widespread assumption that the doctor both knew best and would always act in the patient's best interest. This, of course, can clash with the first principle of respect for autonomy, especially when aiming at patients' welfare may involve decision. Yet the principle of beneficence draws on the long standing "moral obligation to act for the patients' benefit, helping them to further their important and legitimate interests, often by preventing or removing possible harms" (Beauchamp, 2019, para. 3). Although most western societies are now wary of untrammelled medical paternalism, it is also true that in other parts of the world, it is very much commonplace.

Classic paternalistic interventions of placebos typically conflict with the principles of respect for autonomy and beneficence. By deceiving the patient, the physician breaches the principle of respect for autonomy since significant and materially relevant information about the intervention is not provided and thus consent is obviated. Moreover, due to the incipient scientific findings of placebo effects, even though promising, a better-regulated approach to the use of placebos is still needed in order to be in compliance with evidence-based medicine (EBM). Therefore, if the issue of beneficence can be satisfied by scientific evidence and translational research, how placebo use can align with respect for autonomy is still problematic. What might that look like? We turn now to the idea of open-label placebo use.

Ethics of placebos and open-label placebos (OPL) in sports

Recently, Colloca and Barsky (2020) defined placebo effects as the effects of patients' positive expectations concerning their state of health. Two things should be considered here. First, their definition does not include deception as a prerequisite for a placebo effect to exist. Secondly, the use of inert/innocuous substances has also been eschewed, because of new discoveries in placebo studies such as the open-label placebo (OLP). Recent contributions to the definition of placebo such as Colloca and Barsky's, suggest the need for a broader conception of the placebo effect, which includes new strategies in contemporary research for understanding placebo effects.

Because the traditional definitions of placebo include deception, placebo effects are considered to work only when patients believe that they are being treated with a real treatment (despite its inert/innocuous status). Recently, however, results have demonstrated that patients can experience placebo effects, such as pain relief, even when knowing they are taking a placebo (Kaptchuk et al., 2020). Despite recent emerging evidence and excitement with OPL findings, it is still too soon to establish the real conditions in which this intervention will not infringe the principle of beneficence itself since translational research and scientific markers are needed. Moreover, concern exists about how explicit information can be conveyed in a manner that will not unethically manipulate patients' understanding and choices (Annoni, 2018; Annoni & Miller, 2016). Finally, the lack of guidance concerning the framing of the informed consent process while managing patient expectations is a concern (Miller & Colloca, 2011).[3]

Conclusion

It is reasonable to assume that the use of placebo in sport medicine has been very widespread. This commonplace assumption is supported by an older medical ethical perspective that placed significant emphasis on the principle of paternalism – acting in the patient's interest – without a broader evaluation of the relations that pertained between respect for autonomy, non-maleficence and beneficence. It may well be that deceptive placebos did more harm than good, though it is unlikely we could ever know this. Given that absence of evidence, and the rising acknowledgement of respect for patient autonomy as a central principle of clinical professionalism, there will be a need to explore further the balance between ethics and efficacy in, for example, the use of open-label placebo. Clearly, the resultant ethical evaluation will benefit from a stronger scientific body of evidence concerning its effects, both negative and positive.

Notes

1 Those necessary conditions are needed for what we have called the "traditional definition" of the placebo effect. However, one can already identify a trend in the literature in avoiding those two. Accordingly, new definitions are designed to avoid the limitations offered by "treatment" and "inert/innocuous" conceptual elements

for a definition of placebo (Colloca & Barsky, 2020). Nevertheless, there is no substantive consensus on the definition of placebo effects in the literature, despite the presence of putative "consensus statements" published in the literature.

2 By affirming that pain is part of (some professional) sports we by no means intend to morally evaluate those sports here. Suffice here to identify those sports and their presence in widely acceptable international competitions.

3 For a greater in-depth analysis of the use of open-label placebos to enhance sport performance, readers are encouraged to read the chapter by Saunders in this book.

References

Ainslie, D. C. (2002). Bioethics and the problem of pluralism. *Social Philosophy and Policy, 19*(2), 1–28.

Alfano, M. (2015). Placebo effects and informed consent. *The American Journal of Bioethics, 15*(10), 3–12.

Annoni, M. (2018). The ethics of placebo effects in clinical practice and research. *International Review of Neurobiology, 139*, 463–484.

Annoni, M., & Miller, F. G. (2016). Placebo effects and the ethics of therapeutic communication: A pragmatic perspective. *Kennedy Institute of Ethics Journal, 26*(1), 79–103.

Beauchamp, T. (2019). The principle of beneficence in applied ethics. In E. N. Zalta (Ed.), *The Stanford Encyclopedia of Philosophy*. https://plato.stanford.edu/archives/spr2019/entries/principle-beneficence/.

Beauchamp, T., & Childress, J. (2019). Principles of biomedical ethics: Marking its fortieth anniversary. *The American Journal of Bioethics, 19*(11), 9–12.

Beedie, C. J., & Foad, A. J. (2009). The placebo effect in sports performance: A brief review. *Sports Medicine, 39*, 313–329.

Bostick, N. A., Sade, R., Levine, M. A., & Steward, D. M. (2008). Placebo use in clinical practice: report of the American Medical Association Council on Ethics and Judicial Affairs. *Journal of Clinical Ethics, 19*(1), 59–61.

Brody, H. (2018). Meaning and an overview of the placebo effect. *Perspectives in Biology and Medicine, 61*(3), 353–360.

Brooling, J., Pyne, D., Fallon, K., & Fricker, P. (2008). Characterizing the perception of the placebo effect in sports medicine. *Clinical Journal of Sport Medicine, 18*(5), 432–437.

Buchanan, A. E. (2011). *Beyond humanity? The ethics of biomedical enhancement.* Oxford University Press.

Camporesi, S., & McNamee, M. (2017). Philosophy of sports medicine. In T. Schramme and S. Edwards (Eds.). *Handbook of the philosophy of medicine* (pp. 741–755). Springer.

Carlino, E., Piedimonte, A., & Frisaldi, F. (2014). The effects of placebos and nocebos on physical performance. In F. Benedetti, P. Enck, E. Frisaldi, & M. Schedlowski (Eds.), *Placebo* (pp. 149–157). Springer.

Colloca, L. (2014). Placebo, nocebo, and learning mechanisms. *Placebo*, 17–35.

Colloca, L., & Barsky, A. J. (2020). Placebo, nocebo, and learning mechanisms. In F. Benedetti, P. Enck, E. Frisaldi, & M. Schedlowski (Eds.), *Placebo* (pp. 17–35). Springer.

Colloca, L., & Benedetti, F. (2005). Placebos and painkillers: Is mind as real as matter? *Nature Reviews Neuroscience, 6*(7), 545–552.

Dixon, N. (2016) Internalism and external moral evaluation of violent sport. *Journal of the Philosophy of Sport*, 43(1), 101–113. https://doi.org/10.1080/00948705. 2015.1115360

Dworkin, G. (2017). Autonomy. *A Companion to Contemporary Political Philosophy*, 439–451.

Edwards, S. D., & McNamee, M. (2006). Why sports medicine is not medicine. *Health Care Analysis, 14*, 103–109.

Evers, A. W., Colloca, L., Blease, C., Annoni, M., Atlas, L. Y., Benedetti, F., Bingel, U., Büchel, C., Carvalho, C., & Colagiuri, B. (2018). Implications of placebo and nocebo effects for clinical practice: Expert consensus. *Psychotherapy and Psychosomatics, 87*(4), 204–210.

Franklyn-Miller, A., Etherington, J., & McCrory, P. (2011). Sports and exercise medicine—specialists or snake oil salesmen? *British Journal of Sports Medicine, 45*(2), 83–84.

Gleyse, J. (2013). The machine body metaphor: From science and technology to physical education and sport, in F rance (1825–1935). *Scandinavian Journal of Medicine & Science in Sports, 23*(6), 758–765.

Grünbaum, A. (1981). The placebo concept. *Behaviour Research and Therapy, 19*(2), 157–167.

Guijarro, C. (2015). A history of the placebo. *Neurosciences History, 2015*(2), 68–80.

Hainline, B., Derman, W., Vernec, A., Budgett, R., Deie, M., Dvořák, J., Harle, C., Herring, S. A., McNamee, M., & Meeuwisse, W. (2017). International Olympic Committee consensus statement on pain management in elite athletes. *British Journal of Sports Medicine, 51*(17), 1245–1258.

Howe, P. D. (2003). *Sport, professionalism and pain*. Routledge.

Hróbjartsson, A., & Norup, M. (2003). The use of placebo interventions in medical practice—a national questionnaire survey of Danish clinicians. *Evaluation & the Health Professions, 26*(2), 153–165.

Huizenga, R. (1995). *You're OK, it's just a bruise: a doctor's sideline secrets about pro football's most outrageous team*. Macmillan.

Hurst, P., Schipof-Godart, L., Szabo, A., Raglin, J., Hettinga, F., Roelands, B., Lane, A., Foad, A., Coleman, D., & Beedie, C. (2020). The placebo and nocebo effect on sports performance: A systematic review. *European Journal of Sport Science, 20*(3), 279–292.

Kaptchuk, T. J., Hemond, C. C., & Miller, F. G. (2020). Placebos in chronic pain: Evidence, theory, ethics, and use in clinical practice. *BMJ, 370*.

Kayser, B. (2020). Why are placebos not on WADA's Prohibited List? *Performance Enhancement & Health, 8*(1), 100163.

Kent, M. (2006). *Oxford dictionary of sports science and medicine*. Oxford University Press.

Kirkwood, K. (2014). What do you mean I wasn't cheating? Testing the concept of cheating through a case of failed doping. *Sport, Ethics and Philosophy, 8*(1), 57–64.

Mahon, J. (2016). *The Definition of Lying and Deception*. https://plato.stanford.edu/ archives/win2016/entries/lying-definition

McNamee, M., & Morgan, W. J. (2015). *Routledge handbook of the philosophy of sport*. Routledge.

Miller, F. G., & Colloca, L. (2011). The placebo phenomenon and medical ethics: Rethinking the relationship between informed consent and risk–benefit assessment. *Theoretical Medicine and Bioethics, 32*, 229–243.

Morgan, W. J. (2009). Athletic perfection, performance-enhancing drugs, and the treatment-enhancement distinction. *Journal of the Philosophy of Sport, 36*(2), 162–181.

Murray, T. H. (2015). Doping and anti-doping: An inquiry into the meaning of sport. In *Routledge handbook of the philosophy of sport* (pp. 315–332). Routledge.

Nixon, H. L. (1992). A social network analysys of influences on athletes to play with pain and injuries. *Journal of Sport and Social Issues, 16*(2), 127–135.

Parens, E. (1995). The goodness of fragility: on the prospect of genetic technologies aimed at the enhancement of human capacities. *Kennedy Institute of Ethics Journal, 5*(2), 141–153.

Parry, J. (1998). Violence and aggression in contemporary sport. In M. J. McNamee & J. Parry (Eds.), *Ethics and sport* (pp. 205–224). Routledge.

Porter, R. (2004). *Blood and guts: A short history of medicine.* WW Norton & Company.

Raja, S. N., Carr, D. B., Cohen, M., Finnerup, N. B., Flor, H., Gibson, S., Keefe, F., Mogil, J. S., Ringkamp, M., & Sluka, K. A. (2020). The revised IASP definition of pain: Concepts, challenges, and compromises. *Pain, 161*(9), 1976.

Russell, J. S. (2005). The value of dangerous sport. *Journal of the Philosophy of Sport, 32*(1), 1–19.

Shea, M. (2020). Forty years of the four principles: Enduring themes from Beauchamp and Childress. *The Journal of Medicine and Philosophy: A Forum for Bioethics and Philosophy of Medicine, 45*(4–5), 387–395.

Suits, B. (2014). *The Grasshopper: games, life and utopia.* 3rd ed. Broadview Press.

Szabo, A., & Müller, A. (2016). Coaches' attitudes towards placebo interventions in sport. *European Journal of Sport Science, 16*(3), 293–300.

Waddington, I., Scott-Bell, A., & Malcolm, D. (2019). The social management of medical ethics in sport: Confidentiality in English professional football. *International Review for the Sociology of Sport, 54*(6), 649–665.

INDEX

Abduction movement 114
Acclimatisation 86
Acetazolamide 89
Active inference 77
Acupuncture 157, 158
Adenosine receptors 41
Adrenaline 60, 139
Alcohol 145, 147
Alkalosis 89, 91
Allergies 16
Altitude 85–96; Hypoxia 86, 88, 91;
    Normoxia 95; Training 36, 158
Amanzio, M. 39
American Psychological Association 147
Amorphine 39
Amphetamines 2, 145
Anabolic steroids 23, 24, 29, 30, 144,
    147, 150
Anchisi, D. 77
Andani, E. 15
Ansdell, P. 30
Anthropology 46, 50
Anti-depressants 101, 102
Anxiety 15–18, 30, 42, 50, 57, 60–65,
    85, 99, 103, 104, 125, 127, 128
Ariel, S. 29
Arousal 27, 41, 50
Arsène Wenger 150
Aspirin 89
Attention 15, 103, 104, 114, 115, 117
Attitudes 146, 148, 172
Australian Institute of Sport 159

Balance 119, 120
Balanced placebo design 3, 80, 106,
    107, 137, 148, 151
Bayes, T. 73
Bayesian brain 72–82
Beauchamp, T. 176
Beecher, H. 2
Beedie, C. 4, 5, 15, 19, 26, 28, 41, 42,
    49, 123, 148, 151, 161
Benedetti, F. 12, 37, 38, 64, 94, 105,
    115
Benjamin Franklin 1, 2
Beta-alanine 27
Bingel, U. 17
Biofeedback 66
Blood transfusion 144
Blumenstein, B. 25
Body image 104
Bottom-up/Top-down 113, 115, 119
Boxing 125, 129, 173
Bradykinesia 14
Brain imaging 16, 34;
    Electroencephalography 34, 40, 42,
    115, 138; Functional near-infrared
    spectroscopy 42; Functional magnetic
    resonance imaging 17, 34;
    Magnetoencephalography 34;
    Positron Emission Tomography 39,
    41
Brain regions 34, 42, 62, 100; Anterior
    cingulate cortex 36, 63; Basal ganglia
    37; Contralateral Rolandic operculum

16; Frontal operculum 17;
Hippocampus 17; Insula accumbens
36, 63; Nucelus accumbens 36;
Posterior insular cortices 17;
Prefrontal cortex 18, 36, 63;
Putamen 39; Striatum 39, 40, 42;
Thalamus 41, 42
Broatch, J. 24
Brody, H. 170
Brooling, J. 174
Buchel, C. 17, 78

Caffeine 4, 23–30, 36, 39–43, 80, 115,
119, 123, 126, 139, 146, 150, 159, 161
Carbohydrate 24, 26, 48, 123, 150, 159
Cardiovascular 14, 92, 96, 139; Blood
pressure 104; Bradycardic 92; Cardiac
output 86; Heart rate 86, 92;
Tachycardia 92; Vasodilation 86
Central governor 67, 93
Central nervous system 37, 47
Cerebral perfusion 92, 95
Chemoreceptors 86
Chiropractic 157
Cholecystokinin 18, 42
Clark, V. 26
Coaching 124, 133, 174
Cocaine 40, 145
Cognition 17, 40, 48, 103, 117, 129
Cold water-immersion 24, 36, 158
Collagiuri, B. 13
Colloca, L. 12, 13, 177
Complementary alternative medicine 66,
156–164, 174
Concussion 157
Confidence 5, 124–128
Corbett, J. 30
Cortisol 18, 60
Conditioning 107, 114, 138, 147, 151;
Definition 7, 12; Partial
reinforcement 13; Pavlovian 39, 107,
134; Preconditioning 12, 13, 15, 17,
29, 37, 38, 77, 79, 89–94, 107, 115,
119
Conscious 7, 12, 26, 46, 49, 60, 61, 63
Cottrell, N. 50
Creatine 4, 126
Cupping 158
Cycling 5, 26, 27, 30, 41, 48, 105, 135,
136, 145, 150, 156, 173

Damasio, A. 46
De la Fuente-Fernandez, R. 39

Deception 58, 66, 133, 135, 152, 162,
169–179
Depression 40, 63, 85, 104
Denis Shapovalov 173
Diazepam 64
Dietary nitrate 126
Distraction 99
Dopamine 34, 36, 39–43, 75, 85, 99,
138
Doping 24, 38, 81, 144–152, 159, 174;
Davis, J. 40; Festina Scandal 145
Duncan, M. 29

Edwards, S. 174
Electric shock 12, 12
Electromagnetic therapy 157
Emotion 11, 13, 40, 57–67, 104, 126,
129, 137, 138; Affect 17; Feelings
48, 61, 63, 103; Mood 60, 104, 128
Endocannabinoid 36, 37, 45, 108;
Receptors 37, 38, 85
Endocrine system 59, 85
Energy expenditure 48
Ernst, E. 105
Erythropoietin 24, 147, 150
Ethics 58, 86, 88, 95, 103, 125, 128,
133, 147, 161–163, 169–179
Evers, A. 170
Evolution 46–48, 50, 51, 59, 60, 61, 73
Expectations 7, 100, 138, 145–147,
161, 177; Beliefs 7, 25, 37, 47, 48,
105, 123, 124, 127, 129, 145;
Modification 105, 107, 108, 123–130;
Verbal suggestions 3, 5, 11, 12, 13,
14, 17–19, 28, 39, 41, 58, 65, 77,
105, 114, 115, 117, 119, 134, 137,
171; Visual cues 16, 18, 105
Exercise 15, 16, 18, 23, 99–109, 123

False feedback 30, 48
Fatigue 8, 11, 16, 19, 26, 30, 40, 46,
47, 48, 64, 81, 93–96, 99, 115, 118,
135, 139; Mental fatigue 40–42
Fear 13
Fentanyl 17
Fight or flight 60
Finasteride 14
Fiorio, M. 117
Flaten, M. 14
Flowers, K. 135
Fluoxetine 40
Foad, A. 26
Football 175

Foroughi, C. 103
Fitts, P. 116–117
Force production 15, 29, 30, 113

Gait 120
Glucose 34
Grahl, A. 78
Grünbaum, A. 170
Guevarra, D. 138
Guijarro, C. 170
Guillot, A. 24

Harry Gallagher 150
Headache 88–89, 92–93, 161
Heroin 145
Homeopathy *see* complementary
    alternative medicine
Homeostasis 46–47, 50, 52, 60, 62, 65
Hope 47
Hulston, C. 26
Human growth hormone 144
Hurst, P. 11, 15, 19, 23–24, 28, 80,
    137, 146, 148

Imagery 66, 125, 127
Immune system 85
Insomnia 88
International Olympic Committee 145,
    173
International Society for Mountain
    Medicine 86
Interoception 62
Irritable Bowel Syndrome 135
Ischemic preconditioning 23–24, 158
Isotonic exercise 16
Itch 16

Kaasinen, V. 41
Kalasountas, V. 29
Kaptchuk, T. 134, 136, 160
Ketorolac 38
Kinesology tape 23–24, 158
Kirsch, I. 7
Knut Jenson 145
Konings, M. 30

Labelling 18
Lactate 26
Lake Louise Score Questionnaire 88
Lane, A. 67
Lavossier, A. 1
Learning 17, 72–73, 117, 119, 151
Ledoux, J. 61

Leg extension 15, 29, 118–119
Levine, J. 36
Lidstone, S. 39
Lindheimer, J. 100, 107
Lung Cancer 15
Luparello, T. 14

Maganaris, C. 24, 29, 147, 150
Marocolo, M. 24
Mayberg, H. 40
McClung, M. 27, 148
McNamee, M. 171
Memory 17, 37
Mental health 96, 101; Mental health
    model 67
Mesmer, F. 1
Mesmerism 1
Michael Johnson 126
Michael Phelps 158
Mind-body dualism 47, 51–52, 72
Mondaini, N. 14
Morgan, W. 67
Morphine 15, 17, 36–38, 115
Motivation 3, 24, 26, 30, 36, 39, 40,
    47, 49, 128, 138
Motor control 14, 40, 113–120
Mountain sickness 88
Mouth rinsing 48

Naloxone 36, 37
National Health Interview Survey 156
Nausea 88, 161
Nervous 30, 125
Neuroticism 14
Noakes, T. 61, 67
Nocebo effect 5, 11–19, 28, 41–42, 95,
    123, 125, 134, 161, 170, 172;
    Definition 5, 11; Side effects 6, 95,
    170
Non-steroidal anti-inflammatory drugs
    37–38

Ojanen, M. 105
Olympic 145, 150, 158
Opioid 17, 34–39, 41, 45, 75, 108
Overtraining 171, 175
Oxford Dictionary of Sports Science &
    Medicine 175

Pacing 30, 47, 80, 129
Panic 18
Parkinson's disease 14, 39, 85, 120
Parkrun 51

Pain 8, 11–12, 15–19, 26, 36, 41, 46, 63, 79, 99, 104, 115–116, 135, 171, 173; Analgesia 36–38, 52; Nocieption 11, 12, 17, 37, 88; Hypoalgesia 12, 13, 16, 18, 77, 107; Tolerance 37–38
Pentagastrin 64
Perceptual illusion 77
Perceived exertion 8, 29, 46–48, 104, 116, 139
Placebo: Active 4, 125; Definition 1, 2, 6, 35, 58; Impure 5; Open label 3, 133–140, 159, 162; Placebo control 1, 2, 4; Sex 13, 16, 139; Sham 24, 39, 107, 118, 171
Placebo effect: Criticisms 3, 45–46, 89; Definition 4, 53, 123, 133, 169–171, 177, 178; Headroom 63, 162; Non-specific effects 2–4, 28; Placebo response vs. effect 4, 104, 170; Responsiveness 8, 13, 27, 53, 67, 160; Self-fulfilling 146; Social 29, 45–53, 100
Pires, F. 26
Planes of motion 120
Pollo. A 15, 29, 119
Pontzer, H. 50
Practitioner-patient relationship 6, 21
Prediction-error 72–82
Pregnancy 18
Probabilistic theorem 73
Proglumide 64
Prostate 14
Protein drinks 158
Psychological skills training 125

Raglin, J. 67
Rafael Nadal 173
Randomised controlled trial 3, 25–26, 100, 104–105, 156, 160, 176; Blinding 4, 27, 102, 158; Demand characteristics 102–103; No treatment control 15, 28, 100–105, 127, 135
Regression to the mean 104
Remifentanil 17
Respiratory system 14, 26, 36, 85–96, 136; Asthma 14; Bronchoconstriction 14, 17; Blood oxygen saturation 86, 89, 92–96; Dypnoea 17; Hyperventilation 86, 88–92; Ventilation 85–86, 88, 92
Rehabilitation 16
Relief 14

Reproductive system 14
Resource allocation 63
Response bias 138
Reward 39
Richard Virenque 150
Rimonabant 38
Ross, R. 24, 150
Rossettini, G. 114
Rossow, L. 136–137
Rozin, P. 19
Rugby 75, 175
Running 15, 25–28, 80, 128–129, 152, 175

Saunders, B. 4, 27, 135, 137–138
Self-efficacy 81, 127–129
Self-esteem 104
Self-talk 48, 66
Sensory 4, 5, 72–73, 81
Serial reaction time task 117–118
Serotonin 40
Sexual side effects 14
Skiing 25, 175
Social facilitation 50
Social learning 5, 13
Sodium bicarbonate 24, 27, 30, 148, 150, 159
Spinal cord 17–18
Sport Medicine 156, 169–179
St Clair-Gibson, A. 67
Stone, M. 30
Strafella, A. 29
Stress 18, 128
Strychnine 145
Subjective bias 104
Superstitions 125
Surgery 14, 135
Swafford, A. 136–137
Swimming 24, 150, 175
Szabo, A. 174

Taekwondo 124
Tennis 24, 173
Terry, P. 67
Thermal stimulation 12–13, 79
Threat 45
Tinnerman, A. 18
Tolusso, D. 28
Transcranial direct current stimulation 118
Transcranial electrical nerve stimulation 14–16, 23–24, 77, 79, 114, 117, 119, 147
Triplett, N. 50

Ultrasound 158
Ultraviolet 5

Vigor 8
Virtual reality 30
Volkow, N. 40

Wager, T. 72
Weightlifting 24, 29, 135, 147, 150

Well-being 101, 120, 159, 163, 175, 177
Williams, E. 30
World Anti-Doping Agency 144, 159

Yoga 157

Zubieta, J. 36